CORONA
Yesterday, Today and Tomorrow

DR V T KRISHNADAS MENON

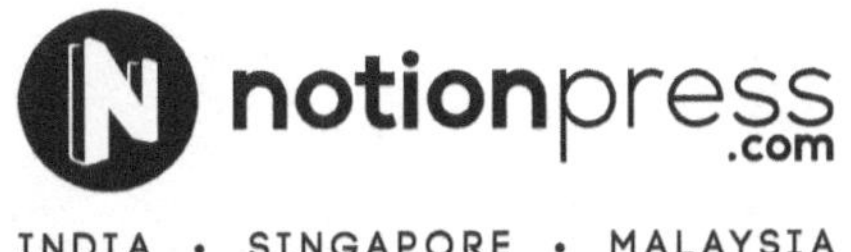

INDIA · SINGAPORE · MALAYSIA

Notion Press

No.8, 3rd Cross Street,
CIT Colony, Mylapore,
Chennai, Tamil Nadu – 600004

First Published by Notion Press 2021
Copyright © Dr V T Krishnadas Menon 2021
All Rights Reserved.

ISBN 978-1-63781-540-3

Dedicated to my late parents
who brought me into
this world and introduced
me to the world of books.

Dedicated also to my wife and daughter
who supported me
in this venture.

CHAPTER 1

As we all know, the world in 2020 is in the grip of the greatest pandemic in recent times. Before going into the story it is essential to know a few terms and a bit of epidemiology. An epidemic by definition is an outbreak of diseases above the expected numbers in a particular geographic area.

A Pandemic on the other hand is an epidemic that has affected several countries.

One of the first reported pandemics of the last century was the Spanish flu caused by H1 NI virus. Although termed as Spanish Flu the first case apparently occurred in Texas, USA. This occurred between 1917 and 1918 during the First World War and was given the name Spanish Flu since Spain was neutral during the War and there was no press censorship of any sort in Spain as it was in many other countries. It was also called Brazilian Flu in Senegal while Brazil called it German Flu and Poland called it Bolshevik disease. The symptoms were fever, headache, cough and cold quite similar to ordinary flu but the only difference was the severity of the spread.

It is reported to have affected 50 million people world wide which is more than the actual numbers who died as a result of the war.

It must be remembered here that medical science had not advanced much as far as the development of vaccines and antibiotics were concerned.

Also it was wartime and countries were divided into their allegiances. The United Nations and World Health Organisation WHO had yet to be formed. Also with war there was little scope for communication both within the country and also across countries.

In British ruled India there were a staggering 10 million deaths.

One of the reasons for its rapid spread across the world was supposedly the World War1.

Most countries sent their soldiers to fight the war the troops were housed in close surroundings in unfamiliar barracks and this led to the rapid spread.

Again when some of them returned from their place of posting they carried the disease with them. Many prisoners of war were released and they returned to their home countries only to bring the virus back with them. Also it was wartime and there was a crowding of the makeshift military hospitals that added to the spread of the disease. Some reports from USA suggested that the virus was present in animals and then mutated and later affected many. There were also reports of some of the early victims staying close to piggeries and it may have possible that the disease may have been contracted from there.

There were apparently 3 waves of the pandemic and it affected countries and regions as far as Alaska and Western Samoa and Australia. Many indigenous people including Inuit tribes of Alaska were almost wiped out. It was said that the King of Spain Alfonso the thirteenth also contracted the disease. The grandfather of US President Donald Trump actually died of this disease.

Again while most countries had a sizeable number of cases China did not seem to have many cases.

Some reports suggested that there was lack of data some reports suggested that the Chinese had developed some resistance to influenza. Some reports suggested that contrary to popular perception it did affect the interiors of China, the data of which is not fully available because most of the data was from major ports of entry. It was suggested that China had this virus earlier too as early as 2015 before it officially become Spanish Flu.

As the disease raged, several measures quite similar to the present measures were introduced. USA for example introduced social distancing norms and fines for coughing or sneezing in public. People were taught cough etiquette. In Japan they introduced face masks which was also introduced in USA.

Staggering of business activity was introduced and so also lockdown. Ban was there for mass gatherings and later on, maritime quarantine was also introduced for many areas. Selective inoculation was also introduced.

The Spanish flu affected about 500 million people world wide roughly one fourth of the world's population at that and a conservative estimate of deaths worldwide was between 17 to 40 million with a possibility that it could even be 100 million. The majority affected were young people.

In British ruled India the deaths numbered between 11 to 17 million which was approximately 5 percent of India's population then. It is said to have arrived in Bombay (old name of Mumbai) in

September 2018 then in October in Madras (old name of present day Chennai) and in November in Calcutta (old name of Kolkata). Bombay alone had an approximate figure of about 11000 deaths. Mahatma Gandhi father of the Nation was one of the well known persons who contracted this disease. Well known Hindi writer Suryakant Tripathi in his memoirs said the Ganga was full of dead bodies that were cremated. Indeed there was supposedly a shortage of firewood due to the vast numbers of bodies that were cremated.

There was no known treatment and most of the treatment was done using aspirin widely available then and also untried home remedies

The next major documented pandemic of influenza that affected India was in the year 1957. This was the H2N2 virus that is supposed to have its origin in Guizhou, China.

Globally 1 to 4 million deaths are said to have occurred. In India this was as a result was primarily through ships carrying passengers from Malaysia. The Indian Government of the day received information on 11th May 1957 that S.S Rajula a passenger ship carrying about 1622 passengers and a crew of 200 that left Singapore and was due to reach a port, Nagapatnam (or Nagapatam as it was called those days) had about 44 passengers who had developed symptoms of influenza including cough fever and cold within a span of 7 days. The ship was diverted to Madras and was put in quarantine. It was found that there were 44 active cases and 7 cases with very high fever. A medical team was sent to examine all the patients and a team from Pasteur Institute Coonoor took the throat swab sample which finally declared it as another strain of influenza A/Asia /57.

4 of the nurses who boarded the ship on 16th got infected on 18th probably making them the first Indian victims of this strain of influenza virus. On 28th May yet another ship SS State of Tamil Nadu which also was arriving from Singapore with 1065 passengers in board was also was carrying 44 passengers who had the virus.

In no time the 4 southern states of Tamil Nadu, Karnataka, Kerala and Andhra Pradesh got hundreds of cases from these 2 ships. At around the same time cases also began to occur in Bombay and Calcutta both of which again had ports. There were also cases of disease among other states not having direct port facilities. It was not possible however to ascertain which was the first case of this outbreak.

In this particular outbreak a higher number of medical and paramedical personnel were involved.

While a sample of the virus from Malaysia was flown into India as early as May 1957 for using it to make a vaccine, actual production of the vaccine at Pasteur Institute started only in January 1958 and by August 1958 the epidemic had ceased to be a major problem and the vaccine was never used.

Among the empirical treatment used was the use of Mandl's paint which was a combination of Iodine and Potassium Ioide and was used locally on the throat. In addition intravenous Intracolloidal iodine also was used

The next major pandemic of modern times was SARS pandemic that occurred first in November 2002 and lasted for about 8 months. Again this originated from China with the first case occurring in Foshan, Guangdong province, China. SARS stood for Severe Acute Respiratory Syndrome syndrome and was caused by Corona virus the same family which among other things also caused the common cold. This affected approximately 8000 persons in 30 countries world wide and it was characterized by a short respiratory illness. It first started in China then quickly spread to Hongkong, USA, Taiwan and several other counties including India. The first case occurred on 16th November 2002 but the index patient died and China did not inform the rest of the world till February 2003. It was then identified as the same virus that occurred in a group of cave dwelling bats. This particular pandemic was numerically much smaller than the previous two in the number of cases. However the case fatality was as high as 11.1 percent. India had only 3 confirmed cases of SARS as per official information. Years later the Chinese said that civet cats which are delicacy in the region could be a possible carrier and the disease may have existed in them before affecting man.

CHAPTER 2

The first reported case of the disease to be known as Covid 19 or Corona occurred in Wuhan city in Huebei province in China on November 19th 2019. The first patient was a 55 year old person from Hubei Province in China. Soon after that case 1-5 cases were reported every week. By December 15th there were 27 cases and by December 20th there were 60 cases. By December 27th there were 180 cases. The World Health Organisation was informed by China country office of World Health Organisation WHO on 31st December. At the point of time the cases seemed to be linked to a seafood market in Wuhan which was subsequently closed in January 1st. On January 7 the virus was identified as N Corona virus or Novel Corona virus or Covid 19.

As early as December a Chinese ophthalmologist Dr Lie Wenliang working at Wuhan Central Hospital sent a message to his medico friends asking them to wear masks and protect themselves and thought the new disease was like SARS. 4 days later he was picked up by the authorities in China who accused him of making false claims. On January 10tth he developed symptoms of cough and fever and was admitted in hospital. He was diagnosed with Corona on January 30th and died on February 7th.

This death shocked the entire scientific community and sent shock bells ringing across the entire world.

Much later yet another virologist from China Dr Li Men Liang who was involved in the outbreak in China fled to USA in April and in September she declared on television from a secret hideout in USA that the virus was actually created in a laboratory in Wuhan, China.

The initial symptoms included fever, breathing difficulty. Later on symptoms began to include diarrhea and anosmia or inability to smell.

However the genomic sequencing of the disease was released only on January 10th 2020.

However that by itself did not cause much concern because many new viruses were being discovered on a fairly regular basis and while some of them were contagious and fatal many of them were localised to their country of origin or at best a few adjoining countries. In recent years Ebola was one such disease that emerged suddenly was very lethal but did not really cause problems beyond a handful of countries.

In the month of January a shut down was imposed for the first time in Hubei province of China which also included Wuhan its main city. In a few days China started reporting hundreds of cases and cases were also reported from Italy, Iran and USA and other countries in South East Asia. On February 3rd the first case of Corona in India was detected. This was a medical student from Wuhan who flew from Kolkata to Kochi on 22rd January after arriving from China the previous day and hailed from Thrissur, Kerala. Soon after the second case also occurred in Kerala and was also in a medical student from Wuhan, China. The third case also was a case of a medical student who travelled also from Kolkata to Kochi also having arrived from China the previous day. Till then the pattern of the disease world wide seemed to be rather unclear. A number of unanswered questions were there.

How did it begin?

Was it spread by bats as some said?

Meanwhile on 30th January the World Health Organisation declared it as a public health emergency of International concern PHEIC but it stopped shy of declaring it as a pandemic.

On March 11th however Corona or Covid 19 was declared as a pandemic

On March 24^d India started its first ever lockdown.

CHAPTER 3

One of the early incidents that took place during Corona was the outbreak on a luxury cruise liner Diamond Princess which was owned by Carnival Cruises. This cruise which began around the time of the Chinese Lunar New Year was a round trip that covered South East Asia starting and ending in Yokohama. This cruise started in Yokohama on 20th January and had 2655 passengers and 1044 crew members from different nationalities. Among its passengers was an 80 year old man from Guangdong, China who flew to Yokohama and boarded the ship despite having a slight cough. He disembarked at Hong Kong on 25th January. The ship left Hong Kong and proceeded to Vietnam, Taiwan and finally to Yokohama its last destination.

Meanwhile on 1st February the person who got off tested positive for the virus and the Hong Kong authorities alerted the authorities in Japan and also the ship authorities. By this time the cruise liner had reached Tokyo Bay, Yokohama and was awaiting instructions.

What were the options available?

The first one was letting all the passengers disembark at Yokohama without doing anything. This would have resulted in several cases in Japan which was due to host the Summer Olympics in a few months. The second option was to allow them to disembark and stay in quarantine in hotels in Yokohama. This would again create a lot of problems.

Another option was to put all of them in flights to their home countries something which would have resulted in introducing infection in almost all countries because the passengers and crew were from all. At this point in time the WHO had not yet declared it to be a pandemic. Finally it was decided to quarantine the ship for a period of 14 days. This was the 15th century age old practice of Cordon Sanitaire. Cordon Sanitaire is a French term meaning building a sanitary cordon around an area so that no infection can reach there.

In the earlier days this involved building a wall or creating new boundaries so that nobody could enter or leave the area. This was effectively used in several countries earlier for outbreaks of Plague, Yellow Fever, Ebola, SARS. This was also the method used in Wuhan with a new terminology namely lockdown.

Medical teams came aboard the ship and on the very first day and screened 31 passengers out of which 10 turned positive. It was a unique situation in that the original passenger had got off the ship 6 days ago and passengers had tested positive now. Now in luxury cruise liners of this sort the majority of passengers are over the age of 60 years many of whom would be having co morbidities and there is a fair mingling of passengers, and passengers and crew members. Also at the time of initial testing the Captain's announcements were not very clear as to why there was a delay in disembarking and why some people were being tested. Quite e a few of the passengers noted that some safety measures had been introduced but they didn't quite grasp the problem they were going to face.

Others who were in the deck found a number of persons wearing HazMat suits and entering the ship. They also saw ambulances parked at the pier. Some of them posted these pictures on Twitter and Instagram and Facebook only to get updated by their online friends that indeed the ship was quarantined. By then the captain had no option but to disclose to the entire ship that the ship was quarantined for 14 days and requested all those with symptoms to get screened. By the end of the exercise about 700 persons had tested positive including crew members and 7 deaths had occurred. All the Corona negative passengers left the ship on 18th. Those who tested positive were sent to various hospitals in Japan for treatment.

In between however several individuals posted videos on YouTube tube asking for help and evacuation. Many appealed to their Presidents and Prime ministers to help them get out of this. USA for instance airlifted about 400 of its citizens to USA before the period of quarantine ended. All together it was chaotic quarantine.

This event led to a lot of discussion. Meanwhile a few claim that quarantine saved about 200 lives others disagreed. One of those who disagreed was noted infectious disease specialist Dr Kentata Iwata of Kobe University who had expertise in both SARS well as Ebola.

He managed to board the ship one day before quarantine and posted some You Tube videos which he was later forced to take down. He noticed that there was free interaction among everybody both those with symptoms and those without symptoms and also those without symptoms.

He famously said that that the cruise ship was a Covid Mill. This was primarily because while persons would be told to stay in their cabins there was always interaction with crew members and others. Common dining and games and dances were there before 4th February but after that it was stopped. However interaction with crew members who brought them food and other essentialities were there leading to more infections. It must be mentioned though that knowledge of the disease was rudimentary at that stage and concepts of social distancing, wearing masks had not come into being. Some others said that this was the world's largest floating Petri Dish. Petri dish is a bowl in which bacteria or viruses are allowed to grow or culture. This is where the virus gets more chance to multiply because of closed confines. Perhaps the last word on this came from a reporter during a briefing by the Health ministry in Japan who asked 'What exactly did the quarantine achieve apart from an extension of 2 weeks?'

CHAPTER 4

Till March though the disease which had developed epidemic forms and affected several countries leading the World Health organisation to label it a pandemic obviously labelling a disease as a pandemic was not easy as it had several economic a and international ramifications

But what was it all about till then?

How was the pattern of disease and the spread? What were the putative risk factors?

At that point of time several theories were put forth and several suggestions came out.

Firstly it was said that it occurred through eating of food from unhygienic Chinese wet markets. Chinese are known for their eating habits and apparently no qualms about eating exotic animals.

Soon videos and visual of some wet markets came out in the media.

A little later came the theory that it was spread through bats very much like Nipah a theory which again was debunked in no time.

Two other animals which were also thought to be the cause of spread were snakes and pangolins both again apparently on the eating list of Chinese.

Clinically what did the picture look like till March. It was basically a disease affecting the upper respiratory tract infection leading to shortness of breath, fever headache running nose. Later on 2 other symptoms were added diarrhoea and anosmia or loss of smell. The last one was considered rather specific but not the only criteria for Covid 19.

While in March almost all countries had been affected there were certain countries that had a huge number of cases and some with relatively very few cases. For example countries with a heavy load in March included apart from China Japan, South Korea, Italy and Iran. In Southeast Asia while the disease was widespread in China, Korea, Japan and Hong Kong it was relatively less in Malaysia, Indonesia and Brunei.

Again Africa which is home to some of the world's oldest and also newest diseases did not seem to have much of a problem.

These led to certain questions which baffled the epidemiologists and public health specialists.

For any communicable disease to be present there had to be what was termed as the epidemiological triad consisting of host agent and environment and interaction between them.

In this case while the agent was known and so also the environment what was not clearly known was the role of the host while man was the host how did he get it infected?

But how did the first person who got infected ever get the infection? How did he transmit the infection?

Epidemiologically in the initial days the disease seemed to more prevalent in certain countries like China, Korea, Japan, Singapore but comparatively less in Malaysia and, Indonesia.

Was it similar to SARS and Nipah?

While Nipah was present very briefly in India in 2018 mainly affecting Kozhikode and Malappuram districts of Kerala there was also a lone case of Nipah in the year 2019 in Ernakulam district Kerala as well.

In the case of Nipah, before the Kerala outbreak there were cases of Nipah from Nadia and Siliguri districts in the Eastern state of West Bengal. Nadia and Siliguri are districts that border Bangladesh where cases were endemic meaning that they were present most of the time. In most of the cases both in West Bengal and Bangladesh there were clear links to fruits and toddy sap which were consumed by bats.

However the origin of Nipah virus was in a place called Kampong Sungei Nipah near the popular tourist town of Port Dickson in Negiri Sembilan in Malaysia. This epidemic first occurred in the nineties and it took a young investigator Dr Kua Bin Chua to unravel the mystery behind it. Apparently all the cases affected the ethnic Chinese only and not the majority Malays. Also it affected only those who worked in pig farms or had contact with pigs. After his pioneering work thousands of pigs were culled in Malaysia and the disease mysteriously stopped in Malaysia. Dr Chua has since migrated to Singapore. In my capacity as a public health specialist formerly with W HO I had sent him a mail as early in March asking about his views and he was extremely gracious to send me a reply which was expectedly guarded and non committal.

Could pigs be a reservoir or intermediate host in Corona cases also?

In the initial days as mentioned above while cases were high in some South Asian countries like China, Japan, Korea, Singapore, Hongkong it wasn't high in Muslim majority countries like Malaysia, Indonesia, Brunei It was also not very high in India, Pakistan, Bangladesh and Gulf countries in March and April.

There was also an outbreak of African swine flu in China that actually ended around October 2019 just before the epidemic started. As a result hundreds of pigs across China were culled.

Was it then due to the Pork eating practices of some of those countries? We still don't know the answer to that.

Again while cases were high in the rest of the world the Indian subcontinent remained relatively free of cases in the initial phases. Was it due to the Subcontinent's practice of washing hands with water after having food in contrast to using tissue paper or chopsticks as was the trend in South east Asian countries?

Again the answer to this is not known. Was it because of the Indian habit of folding hands and saying Namaste as opposed to the usual shaking of hands vin the rest of the world?

Another theory was that while most South East Asian counties did use Airconditioning or Aircon both in homes and offices, in Indonesia, Malaysia and Brunei which had more natural cover. They also used fans and minimised the use of Airconditioners.

Again while the African subcontinent has been the traditional home for several diseases in case of Corona it had relatively fewer cases in the beginning.

What was that due to?

Was it that Africa with a high prevalence of vector borne diseases like Malaria had some sort of immunity to Corona.

.Or was it that the practice of using chloroquine against malaria conferred some degree of immunity against Corona as well. It may be worth pointing out that hyroxychloroquine a derivative of chloroquine was thought to have prophylactic effects against Corona? Again this question does not have any proper answer.

Another theory that was discussed was whether vaccination with BCG the vaccine used against Tuberculosis conferred some level of immunity. In the case of India which has a high proportion of cases of tuberculosis cases compared to the rest of the world almost everybody except those above 60 been immunized against Tuberculosis. So in some uncertain way is it giving rise to some sort of immunity.

Or was it that simply enough testing was not being done since most African countries did not have Corona testing kits in the initial phases.

This was disease that affects the respiratory tract mainly and while it is similar to the common cold and a host of other diseases not every case of cold or cough had to be Corona or Covid. And therein lies the first problem.

For a person to be labelled as a Corona case he had to be tested. The Gold standard for testing was the RTPCR or Reverse Transcriptase Polymerase Chain Reaction test. This test during the initial days was hard to come by because there were fewer test kits available Moreover many cases of Corona were there which never had symptoms and hence were never diagnosed. These were either subclinical infections or carriers with potential to spread the disease. However they went undetected as they did not have any symptoms.

Apart from direct droplet infection as through sneezing or coughing did fomites also play a role in this. Fomites are basically inanimate objects that can be the prospective place where the virus can survive and replicate. Studies done later said that the virus can survive for days or even months on metal wood and other surfaces. The first patients were air travellers and it possible that fomites included the aircraft seats, the handles, the over head luggage racks. More importantly in the airport setting was the possible presence of virus on airport trolleys, luggage belts, wash room doors X ray screening counters, and Coffee shops, duty free shops all of which had the potential to have fomites

CHAPTER 5

In January the province of Hubei in China declared its lockdown which was the first anywhere in the world. All flights, trains and other forms of public transport were banned People were advised to stay indoors

In March after the World Health Organisation declared it a pandemic all countries had a lockdown. By the time it was declared a pandemic almost all countries had cases and most of the cases had a travel history from China. However there were several cases that had no travel history either and were a result of local spread.

In the case of South Korea for example the initial cases had a travel history from China but majority of cases were due to some events which resulted in free intermingling. However one of the main events was due to a function at a church from where the disease spread like wildfire.

In Malaysia also the rise of cases was small to start with but eventually there was a spurt of cases due to a religious event in Petaling Jaya, Selangor by a religious organisation Tablighi Jamaat that led to a rise in cases there.

Italy and Iran were 2 other countries as different as chalk and cheese which also had huge spikes in cases. In the case of Italy again while the travellers from China were the initiators there was also local spread. To make matters worse Italy also saw a number of deaths mainly among the elderly population who had severe co morbidities like diabetes, hypertension. One of the reasons that was attributed was apparent segregation of old persons in nursing homes.

A somewhat similar pattern unfolded in USA too where number of cases and fatalities kept rising. The newspapers were full of obituaries of persons who had died of Corona.

By this time the World Health Organisation started giving daily briefings and some clarity came over the steps that need to be taken.

One of the first and most important steps was that of social distancing which actually meant physical distancing. It was said that stating 2 meters away from anyone else greatly reduced the risk of spread.

This would literally keep the virus at arms length. Yet another guideline was regarding sanitation. Apart from using soap and water every time people were encouraged to sanitise their hands every time. There were also sanitising machines that sprayed the sanitising liquid all over.

Yet another involved the use of Personal protection equipment or PPE. While the definition of full PPE remained ambiguous at the beginning it actually meant use of masks. Again as far as masks were concerned there were controversies about the types of masks to be used. It was broadly agreed that N95 masks without respirator valves were considered the best. This had been earlier used during the SARS pandemic also. This was followed by layered cloth masks and ordinary surgical masks. There were also criteria for certain categories like health workers support staff who in addition to N95 masks also had to wear Shields, HazMat suits and gloves and boots

CHAPTER 6

So how was the disease progressing till the month of March. One would need to gave a travel history to China or be in close contact with someone with a travel history to China

So does the flight lasting for a few hours increase the chance of spread of virus. Or more precisely did the chance of travelling in a closed air conditioned space for more than 1 hrs increase the chance of spread. The answer to that was not known. Alternatively what are the chances of getting infected by travelling in a close air conditioned environment like a plane for 2 hours as opposed to a train journey taking say 12 hours or more with approximately 70 passengers (approximately one third that of a international flight) in a non-air conditioned compartment. Once again the answer to that is not known.

Again within what distance can a infected person transmit the disease. In other words if a person is in seat number 1 on a flight what are the chances that he will transmit it to someone sitting in row no 30 for example assuming that there is no other contact between the two either during boarding or disembarking? What are the chances of that infected person in seat Number 1B affecting those sitting say in seat number 1 A or 1C.

Again the answers are not known with clarity.

What if he uses the wash room in the plane or the airport lounge which are also used by co passengers (in the second example of airport wash rooms the other users need not be from the same flight). Once again these answers are not very clear or convincing.

So how did countries respond to it While the WHO declared Corona as pandemic on March 11th many countries already had hundreds of cases as on that date. However at that particular point the Indian subcontinent, Gulf countries, African countries seemed to have much lesser cases as compared to Europe USA, Far East where the disease was raging.

What could have been the cause of this rather lesser number of cases in the initial phases. Was it due to lack of testing either because of lack of information or lack of kits or a combination of both?

Or was it that unlike persons from Europe, USA who eat using fork and spoon and in case if South East Asian counties who use chopsticks most others use their hands and wash it with soap and water as compared to the others who just wipe their hands on tissue paper.

This may have been possible but in a few weeks all countries started having huge number of cases.

CHAPTER 7

One of the earliest and most effective things that was done was quarantine. The word quarantine meant keeping a person in possible contact with a suspected case in a separate place for such time as the longest incubation period of the disease. It was different from isolation in that in isolation the person was actually confirmed with the diseases and could be in isolation in hospital or at home for very mild cases.

In the beginning when the cases were a trickle in India, quarantine was a relatively easy affair. Persons coming in the same flight as a infected case were put in quarantine in designated quarantine centres some of which were free. In due course once the cases piled up quarantine became a very big issue. Even as Indian Prime Minister Narendra Modi reviewed the situation just before lockdown and asked the states about their preparedness for the lockdown most states said they were ready. Kerala went a step ahead and said that they had identified about 2 lakh beds for quarantine a claim that was unfortunately belied a few weeks later. While in the initial days, quarantine was in specially designated camps as mentioned above there were some criteria to be met. There had to be minimum distance of 3 meters or more between beds in such a case. Also there had to be attached toilets. As the number of cases increased persons were given a choice either a paid quarantine for 14 days at certain designated quarantine centres or unpaid quarantine at the persons home. A total of 14 days in a hotel designated for quarantine would cost about Rs 30000 rupees at the bare minimum or about 450 dollars approximately and nobody would be going for this unless there are compelling circumstances at home like say an aged elder or a young child who would be at risk if the person decides to quarantine himself there. Also that place would necessarily have to have a separate attached wash room for the quarantined person. It was also observed that many of those quarantined came from lower income groups and did not have provision for attached bathrooms in their homes. This was particularly true of blue collar workers in Gulf countries. The onus of quarantine was actually on the health staff. A health worker on getting information about the person who tested positive was supposed to inform the person about quarantine and what to do and what not to do. The health worker was also asked to verify if the person had quarantine facilities in his house meaning a separate room with attached bath.

While some states like Karnataka introduced stamping of quarantine persons and Apps to detect quarantined persons, many others did not. In quite a few cases persons in quarantine were seen moving freely. Although the health staff was supposed to make phone calls to the person under quarantine as also that by a social worker or psychologist what was significant was that the calls were made but the persons often used to go outside before during or after the call and there was no way of knowing for the health staff.

Also while neighbours would be knowing about Corona positive cases and those family members in quarantine, what they would not be knowing about someone who is in quarantine because he had an office colleague who was positive or travelled from outside the state or country. In these cases the list was with the concerned health department. To be fair there were some genuine cases for the quarantined person moving around. This was mostly if he had some non Corona ill bedridden patients in his house like for example aged parents or a nearing term pregnant wife or small children. In such a case who would go to do errands?

There were several other problems related to quarantine many of which were mental. Many in quarantine felt very stressed out and in many cases there was initial stigmatisation among the neighbours regarding quarantine. It was as though the person had committed a heinous crime. A dedicated team of psychological counsellors in Kerala would ring up those in quarantine on a daily basis to assess their mental status and also to reassure them.

As part of its awareness campaign all mobille companies and state owned Bharat Sanchar Nigam Limited BSNL started social messaging while waiting for the receiver to pick up. This obviously lead to greater awareness but it had one major drawback. During an emergency even if one called the number for ambulance one was stuck with this message leading to loss of valuable time. Even after 9 months this somewhat irritating caller tune had not stopped.

Another major message was that of social distancing and hand sanitization.

While most places were closed even after lockdown was lifted some restaurants were open with restrictions keeping seats vacant and maintaining the distance. All these places had a sanitizer at hand also. And while many had some sort of entry book where the visitors had to enter their names and phone numbers.

In most cases it was just a formality with nobody really checking and many not writing their phone numbers. The idea behind noting phone numbers was that should anybody become positive and his travel history be traced then this could help in contact tracing.

Another feature was the use of hand held No Touch thermometers. Again while persons were scanned in several cases the records were not kept. In some housing societies in Mumbai for example a record was kept by the security personnel who alerted a resident if there was any rise in temperature.

One of the major problems in Corona was the issue of sudden respiratory distress. Usually any shortage of oxygen or hypoxia characterised by breathlessness which actually serves as a warning. However in case of Corona due to to a cytokine storm which meant that cytokines inflammatory markers of the disease were related in large numbers particularly during sleep often led to what is called Silent Hypoxia.

One way of knowing of knowing if one is having hypoxia is by knowing one's oxygen saturation which in normal circumstances should be round 94 percent or above. The best way if knowing this was by using a portable battery operated pulse oximeter which would give reading once a finger is placed under it. Depending on their quality these were priced from as low as Rs 800 to Rs2000. Many brands also became available online. Some of the cheaper ones however started giving false results. In some of these putting a pencil instead of the finger lead to similar results. Many household started buying these pulse oximeter(genuine) particularly for those in the vulnerable age group.

CHAPTER 8

One of the biggest issues in this pandemic has been the role of China.

Some persons are of the opinion that this is a man made epidemic which later grabbed international attention and was declared a pandemic only after 3 months in March. Many countries are of the view that WHO also stepped in late declaring it as a pandemic only after 3 months in spite of several countries reporting cases. It may be worth recalling that the first documented case occurred in December 2019 and Hubei province in China first declared lock down only on January 23rd Later countries like Italy declared a lockdown. Most countries including India declared a lockdown only after the WHO declared it as a pandemic.

It may be noted here that WHO authorities did not get enough cooperation from the Chinese authorities in the beginning of the epidemic that is around December and January. While Hubei province had one of the longest lockdowns ever thanks to the sheer number of cases there what was surprising was that cities like Beijing and Shanghai did not have that many cases

The first reported cases of the disease to be known as COVID-19 occurred in Wuhan, Hubei province, in late December 2019. China released the genomic sequence of the virus on Jan 10, 2020,

Wuhan was placed under a strict lockdown that lasted for a total of 76 days. Public transport was suspended. Soon afterwards, similar measures were implemented in every city in Hubei province. Across the country, thousand of checkpoints were established at major public transport hubs. School re-openings after were delayed and population movements were severely curtailed. Dozens of cities implemented family outdoor restrictions, which typically meant that only one member of each household was permitted to leave the home every couple of days to collect necessary supplies. In no time China had managed to test 9 million people for SARS-CoV-2 in Wuhan. It set up an effective national system of contact tracing. By contrast, the UK's capacity for contact tracing was overwhelmed soon after the number of cases increased there. China also increased production of clinical gowns and surgical masks. Moreover, the Chinese readily adopted mask wearing.

Compliance with mask wearing was very high compared to other countries like USA

Being a very strict nation rules were much easier to enforce here. There were none of the protests seen in other countries including USA and India. Loudspeakers rebuked Chinese citizens who were not following the rules. In contrast many sporting events were held in USA with thousands of spectators were held before it was declared a pandemic.

On Feb 5, 2020, Wuhan opened three so-called Fangcang hospitals. These were temporary hospitals established in public venues like, exhibition centres and were used. Another 13 would be started later. The hospitals were established within public venues such as stadiums and exhibition centres to isolate patients with mild-to-moderate symptoms of COVID-19. Patients who started to show symptoms of severe disease were quickly transferred to conventional hospitals.

The network of Fangcang hospitals, which held 13 000 beds, meant that patients with COVID-19 did not have to isolate at home, which reduced the risk of family members becoming infected. By March 10, 2020, the Fangcang hospitals were no longer needed. At around the same time, the focus of China's countermeasures shifted from controlling local transmission to preventing the virus from taking hold as a result of imported cases. Those who entered the country were tested and quarantined.

There were also other measures like sanitising the streets and high rise buildings using huge machines

By the time WHO declared it a pandemic China apparently had stopped reporting cases

While studies done in China on the Corona epidemic have to taken with a large pinch of salt one study calculated that the public health actions undertaken by China between Jan 29 and Feb 29 may have prevented 1·4 million infections and 56 000 deaths.

In August, Wuhan hosted a huge pool party and showed the world that Wuhan had become normal

CHAPTER 9

Till March the disease was looking eerily like SARS and Nipah. While for SARs the initial agent was supposed to be pigs and pig products and occurred only to people who ate pork later cases occurred in persons who had never been abroad or ever been in touch with pigs or pork products.

This was quite similar to the SARS epidemic in its early days. Most of the hard hit countries had their first cases as a result of travel from China However in no time the number of cases that had no travel history to China also started rising. While countries like South East Asian countries South Korea, along with Europe and USSA had large numbers the African continent was not really showing in large numbers. To start with probably there were not enough tests done as testing equipment was in short supply in the early days. However unlike other countries fewer persons from Africa would ever go to China for tourism, business or studies. The other aspect was regarding the relative immunity which African persons may have got due to being the malaria endemic zone. It is difficult to comment on this hypothesis but it must be remembered that India too had few cases till March and it was thought that India too was like Africa. Later India had a massive increase in cases and became the second most affected country after USA

After WHO declared a pandemic most countries across the word declared a lockdown PM Modi also declared a lockdown for India. Till then the cases from India were much less and confined mainly to International passenger. The first case of Corona was a medical student hailing from Thrissur, Kerala who arrived from Wuhan just before lockdown was declared. She managed to get on a train to Kumming and later boarded a flight to Kolkata on 23rd and came from Kolkata to Kochi on 24th January the 2nd and 3rd cases of Corona also were young medical students who came in similar fashion from Kumming to Kochi via Kolkata. After that a few cases were reported chiefly from Delhi and Kerala

Kerala which has a very good track record in health managed to restrict itself to 3 cases till March when a family hailing from Pathanamthitta district arriving from Italy hid the information about their travel and they were traced only when some of their neighbours were admitted to hospital with symptoms and were tested positive. A contact tracing was done and subsequently these cases were detected. Other early cases reported in India were also from persons who had returned by air from other countries.

CHAPTER 10

What were the symptoms of Corona or Covid 19. The commonest symptoms according to WHO and Centre for disease control USA are fever, dry cough, fatigue Relatively rare symptoms were diarrhea, anosmia and loss of smell. Most of these symptoms occurred a few days after getting the infection. While cough and fever and fatigue and breathlessness were clinical features of Corona they were also present in a number of other diseases.

Not all cases of fever and dry cough with fatigue were due to Corona. The key to diagnosis was obviously testing for virus. Here the RTPCR was the most accurate test while the Rapid Antigen test or RAT was cheaper and gave results much earlier. In a large number of cases the symptoms did not warrant much to seek an early testing and many consulted doctors who have given them antibiotics like Azithromycin or 3rd generation Cephalosporins and cough syrups

There was also this so called hypoxia which essentially meant that a sudden drop of oxygen without any warning symptoms. This was particularly happening in elderly patients mainly during sleep.

There were also lung changes that could be seen through CT scans or Computerized Scans. Most of them showed fibrosis of the lungs.

As the disease evolved some more things came to light. There was the Post Covid syndrome in which a person suffering from Covid became better and tested negative and after a few days suddenly lost his life This happened to quite a few persons including some well known personalities. Apparently the presence of a Covid negative test was not enough to reverse the long term damage which this virus did to the lungs

While it was not a self limiting disease universally the key to diagnosis was early testing.

The next important thing was Contact Tracing. This was basically to find out who were the contacts of the person. This was usually based on the recall history of the person who turned positive. During the initial days when cases were in just tens and hundreds it was a rather easy job. Nevertheless there were contacts of more than 1000 persons for some affected persons. An NRI in Kerala for example on arrival visited his relatives both on his side and his wife's side and also took part in social functions like marriages, funerals, visited malls. This was not an uncommon phenomenon particularly for Keralites who would be coming to their homeland after 1 or in many cases 2 years from Gulf countries where they worked. While upto a point contact tracing was feasible it was not possible to find out who all attended the marriage or visited the mall or attended the funeral In such cases the district authorities used the media including social media to ask the public to fill in the gaps. Posts were made on Social Media like Facebook and Whats App saying that Mr A visited X Mall on 16th April between 4 pm.to 9pm and requesting all those who were in the mall at that time to come forward and identify themselves and contact the district medical officer or his office.

Many did come forward but many did not do so for avoiding the hassles of quarantine. In later days all visitors to commercial establishments including malls had to enter their phone numbers in a register and also sanitise themselves before entering the mall. However for all practical purposes once the number of cases started increasing this register was just having a cosmetic value as hardly anyone was being called based on the entries in the register

CHAPTER 11

Who were the persons at risk?

While initially it was air travelers particularly those with a travel history to Chins a later it found that the severity was more in those with co morbidities like diabetes hypertension, coronary heart disease, chronic kidney or liver disease and those immunocompromised including those on chemotherapy and taking steroids

It was also found that the mortality rate was higher among the elderly population who by the very nature of the group had co morbidities. As a consequence senior citizens above the age of 65 or 70 were forbidden from going outside. But in a country like India what was to be done in a situation where the elderly parents were alone but children were not staying with them. In most of these case the respective governments rose to the occasion and arranged for their provisions, medical care and other such care. Also helpful neighbours and several organizations also came forward to help them. The problem for the senior citizens was of keeping them indoors. Most senior citizens were in the habit of taking a walk or going to the temple or church or mosque before Covid times. However with no religious place open and restrictions in place most have to be confined to walking in their home, reading newspaper and books and watching television

Surprisingly and thankfully the children been spared of this disease for reasons unknown. There are no reports of mothers dying due to this and thousands of deliveries have occurred during Covid times and there have no documentation of mother to child transmission.

The question that arises then is why are schools closed if it doesn't affect children much? The answer to that lies in the fact that children can mix around freely in school and can in turn bring the infection home thereby jeopardizing the other family members particularly the senior citizens.

Another obvious high risk group was health care workers. Their proximity to patients with or without proper PPE made them at high risk for the infection. Across the globe thousands of health care workers have been affected and several others have died due to this. In India also this has unfortunately been the same pattern and nurses as also senior doctors and nurses have lost their lives to this illness.

A slight lowering of guard and the virus was here. While many doctors doing independent practice have completely stopped going to their clinics some are still continuing to do so.

Many others have resorted to doing telemedicine using apps like What's App, Google Pay. Many doctors including young doctors as well as senior doctors have lost their lives dealing with the pandemic Many were admitted in hospitals and were on ventilators for a long time before succumbing to this disease.

Apart from senior citizens, persons with co morbidities and health care workers another large group affected has been other front line workers like the police who probably contract it as part of the duty In addition after getting the infection it is easier transmitted among their camps. Many such camps of police, Central Reserve Police force, or CRPF, Border security force BSF have been thus affected.

Similar is the case of inmates of old age homes, convents and seminaries where people are cloistered in close confines. Hundreds of cases from these places have been reported

One of the major problems in the disease is the presence of the so called cytokine storm leading to full fledged Acute respiratory distress syndrome ARDS. Cytokines are nothing but inflammatory markers However in case of Corona they ate released in extremely huge numbers leading to Acute respiratory distress syndrome. This in turn lead to lack of oxygen a condition called hypoxia. The problem with this hypoxia was it came often without any symptoms like difficulty in breathing. This gave it the term silent hypoxia. This silent hypoxia apparently affected elders and those with comorbidities

CHAPTER 12

China which had the first and maximum number of cases rapidly brought the number of cases down. How was this possible. The the province of Hubei enforced a strict lock down from January 23rd that lasted for 76 days. In a country like China it was easy to enforce the lockdown much more effectively than several other countries including USA and India.

Apart from enforcing lockdown they also ensured strict adhering to social distancing norms and wearing of personal protective equipment like masks, and gloves. They also tried unconventional treatment methods like combination of antiviral and anti HIV medicines which would appear to have worked. They also did use traditional Chinese medicine or TCM which was given to roughly half the affected population. They also successfully sanitized the streets and buildings using huge machines spraying disinfectant. Apparently that also seemed to have worked. China also built hospitals in record time. These hospitals called Fangcang hospitals were actually temporary structures built in places like stadiums and other public places where those mildly ill could be attended to so that the hospitals which were flooded with both COVID-19 and Non COVID patients don't burst at the seams. Apart from that it also ensured that those persons with mild symptoms don't self isolate at home thereby potentially being at risk to other family members

These moves made by China brought to down the infection rate rapidly and by the time the infection picked up in other countries China's figures showed a down slope. By August the disease had become almost non-existent in China and the city of Wuhan which bore the initial brunt of the epidemic hosted a huge pool party with no restraints and without social distancing. This was a message to the world that China had become normal

IN USA there was a totally different picture. The epidemic had reached enormous proportions and hospitals were swarmed with patients. There was also an apparent shortage of ventilators. However President Donald Trump first brushed aside the epidemic saying it was just like the common flu which also affects thousands every year in the USA and there are quite a few deaths. He was also one of the persons who refused to wear masks even as his principal medical advisor Dr Antony Fauci pleaded for the same. Trump kept ridiculing the use of masks though deaths started mounting and cases reached millions. And while the US system of federalism allowed states to make their own laws regarding health, many states refused to accept social distancing norms and wear masks. In many states the anti maskers hit the street and went to tourist spots like beaches. To make matters worse the death of a black man at the hands of a white police officer and the subsequent protests and marches made things even worse. By then USA had almost hit election time and still Trump was defiant.

By then he had started calling Corona the China virus and had blamed China for the spread of the virus. He also blamed the World Health Organization for not informing the rest of the world and in a drastic move stopped funding to WHO. He also stopped trade relations with China on a majority of items and put a higher tax tariff on them. By the time elections were announced and Joe Biden and Kamala Harris were named as the Democratic pair to challenge Trump and Vice President Mike Pence the disease was spreading rapidly. However while Biden and the rest of democrats wore masks Trump steadfastly refused and even in his rallies and conferences was regularly seen without them. On one of his last meetings on the White House lawns a number of very important persons contracted the disease including many White House staff and a few days later Trump himself became positive.

His face-offs with his principal Health advisor Dr Anthony Fauci a distinguished academic and co editor of the famous book Harrisons's Principles of Internal Medicine had become interesting and more comical day by day. While Fauci advocated use of masks Trump negated him

In fact in one of his last campaign meetings he declared that Fauci with whom he had a lot if differences in opinion would be sacked if Trump was re elected.

Even as Trump was declared positive he was shifted to hospital. The entire world waited with bated breath.

What if something had to happen to Trump rendering him unfit on election day?

Would the elections have to be postponed?

Would the Republicans chose another candidate or would America go through perhaps its greatest ever constitutional crisis? Even as the media and the world was discussing this Trump tweeted saying he is back and while he posted

1 photo wearing a mask the next photo showed him removing his mask and waving to his supporters

He had been given an experimental drug which worked remarkably and put back on his feet in the shortest possible time. There were just a few days to election and Trump did not waste any time however by self isolation any further. In contrast his opponent Joe Biden constantly wore masks and criticised Trump for not doing so Trump was also criticized for getting access to exclusive treatment which the average American would never get. In one of the most polarized bitterly fought elections which was quite close Trump lost and one of the factors that many attribute in his loss was the way he handled the Corona situation. Presently USA has over 19 million cases and more than 3.3 lakh deaths due to Corona

In UK there was a slightly different picture.

Very early into the pandemic a 94 year old Queen Elizabeth and her consort Prince Philip moved from Buckingham palace to Windsor castle a rather smart move. Around the same time Prince Charles became one of the early high profile persons to test positive although asymptomatic and went into isolation. The principal scientific advisor to Prime Minister Boris Johnson, Sir Henry Vallance talked about herd immunity saying that as more persons got effected herd immunity would protect them. Herd immunity was a term that usually referred to a substantial percentage of the population getting immune through vaccination thereby protecting the others also. This was particularly true of tetanus and other diseases where vaccination coverage was not necessarily 100 percent but hovered in the range of 90 percent but that was enough to confer herd immunity.

The problem with this herd immunity concept was that there was no vaccine yet for this condition and for herd immunity to occur through natural infection about 80 percent of the population would have to get the infection So in country with say 100 million population about 80 million persons would have to get affected. With a death rate of about 1 to 3 percent that would work out 8 lakh to 24 lakh deaths die to Corona something which was just not acceptable.

In a short time UK faced a number of cases in its first wave with the numbers including plenty of health care workers.

Prime Minister Boris Johnson himself had to be admitted into a hospital ICU and spent a few anxious days there. He recovered after a few days and profusely thanked the National Health

Service for the wonderful work they had done. By this time the concept of herd immunity also went for a toss and the Government brought in all steps to stop the epidemic Schools colleges shops and establishments were closed and persons were told to exercise inside their homes instead of outside. Pubs and salons also were closed. Senior citizens were also told to stay indoors as also children. Apparently these measures worked while till around late September when the region started showing a second wave although lockdown had been lifted. UK was forced to declare a second lockdown in the month of November ending in 3rd December. It was later extended till the end of December. There was however bad news for UK as initially 2 and later another mutant strain of the virus had surfaced. Both these strains were more contagious than the original one although their virulence was not known fully. It was also not known if the vaccines that were being developed or being used had any effect on this new strain. Another mutant strain had been also found in South Africa which like UK was experiencing its new wave of infections. Yet another mutant strain had also surfaced in Nigeria. The announcement of the mutant strain led to the suspension of flights to and from UK from several countries. Moreover screening procedures intensified for all those who arrived in other countries just before the suspension of flights. To make matters worse it was Christmas season Moreover UK was supposed to break away from the European Union by 31ˢᵗ December. As on Christmas day UK had over 2 million cases with over 70000 deaths

Brazil was another country in the news for very wrong reasons. Its president Bolsarano was another person like President Trump who underestimated the virulence of the virus. He was a person who was in favour of keeping businesses open and also never advocated social distancing, hand washing or wearing a mask Much like Trump he fired his health minister over his attitude towards Corona. Even when President Bolsarano and half his cabinet was affected he refused to wear a mask. He also openly refused to take vaccine either. As on Christmas day Brazil has 7.i million cases and nearly 2 lakh deaths.

The European countries too had roughly the same story as UK. Italy for instance got hit very early on and regions like Lombardy in the northern part of Italy were the worst hit. In Italy a distinct pattern occurred. Majority of the persons infected and who died in nursing homes or elder care centres. These were persons who lived together with people of the same age group and who also had food together and also interacted with others. Due to the pandemic many of them were denied health care as the normal visiting doctor would not come or could not come. Moreover hospitals would also be not admitting such patients generally. This saw a sort of desperation. Many resorted to prayers while others just became fatalistic. As a report suggested, nursing homes were like besieged castles where nobody was allowed to enter or go out. Also most residents never wore masks nor practiced social distancing. Again there were very few tests conducted for them and for those who tested positive there was some slight resistance to getting hospitalized. Some did not like to get admitted in an unfamiliar hospital surrounding for a condition which may prove fatal. Another issue that clouded the minds of these elders was regarding funerals. Many of them though not fully scared of dying were however loath to have a funeral in which even family members would be absent thanks to Covid protocol. Till May. Italy saw more than 30000 deaths second at that time only to USA and Spain. Presently it has crossed 2 million cases with over 70000 deaths. One of the enduring sad images of Corona was that of Pope Francis delivering his Easter Homily all alone in the near empty Saint Peter's Square in Vatican.

One country that received bouquets and brick bats for its handling of the Corona crisis was

Sweden. Sweden with a population of 10 million got its first patients not from China but from families vacationing in the Alps. Sweden never had any lockdown and instead the government went ahead with its idea of herd immunity.

They instead tried to do social distancing and work from home.

However schools were kept open and reports suggest that multiple outbreaks did occur although testing was not done. The idea behind keeping schools open was apparently to allow herd immunity to develop through natural infection something that never really happened.

One of the major issues in Sweden was lack of testing. By extension there was also lack of contact tracing that is finding out who all were the persons in likely close contact.

Initially the figures of Sweden began to stun the world. In spite of no lockdown the number of cases was much less. Indeed it was truly amazing. Maybe the herd immunity concept was working very well after all. Some weeks later another picture came out this time the case fatality rate. As on Christmas day the total number of cases were over 3.96 lakhs with over 8000 deaths.

The very same media that were the biggest fans of the Sweden model became its biggest critics.

A closer look found that the majority of patients who died were elders particularly in old age homes. Many died without getting admitted to hospitals. There was also a triage policy which actually was looking at deaths and was trying to save persons without co morbidities thereby leaving the elders and those with co morbidities to find for themselves.

A recent survey also showed that many Swedes are not in favour of vaccination either and are preferring to acquire herd immunity by getting infected.

In Africa mention must be made of 2 countries which varied vastly in their number of Corona case.

On the one hand there was Nigeria with a population of about 206 million which till December had just over 81000 cases with 1243 deaths. This was a truly remarkable achievement for a country with a large population. On the other hand South Africa with a much smaller population of 59 million had nearly 1 million affected with over 26000 deaths. What contributed to this vast difference in the numbers needs to analyzed fully. Very recently South Africa has reported a new mutant strain of the virus that is more contagious.

In Gulf countries which are generally more stringent in their health regulations the picture was different. Saudi Arabia was the first off the block by stopping Umrah the second most important pilgrimage to Mecca after Haj. Unlike Haj, Umraah can be done at anytime and not just during a particular time of the year.

In a first of its kind the Saudi authorities sealed and sanitized the holy Kaaba, something which had never been done beforehand. Haj was also cancelled for this year. Kuwait which had a spurt of cases in the initial days closed down its airport and declared a lockdown much before Corona was declared a pandemic. Only supermarkets were open and practices like temperature screening, hand sanitization, social distancing were adopted. In UAE also lockdown was declared and while it was there, authorities there sanitized the entire streets of UAE. All establishments were closed as also parks and other places of entertainment. The government there also introduced Apps for quarantining persons. Apart from that massive testing facilities were introduced. UAE also introduce Drive In Kiosks where one could go for testing. While initially tests were costly and perhaps not affordable particularly for the migrant blue collar worker later the rates were reduced. UAE being a small country where the laws are enforced very strictly was a success story as far as Corona is concerned. Similar was the condition in other Gulf countries.

Singapore which again had a number of cases in the initial phases quickly moved in with measures to control the spread.

It was found that majority of cases belonged to migrant workers staying in dormitories and the number of cases of Singapore citizens or permanent residents were much less.

This was in spite of having a fairly high elderly population. Lockdown was imposed and food and other essentials were brought to those who need it particularly those in the dormitories.

Extensive contact tracing was done to find out where all the cases had visited prior to getting infected. These included malls and departmental stores like the famous Mustafa departmental stores and all those who visited these places were also tracked. In Singapore too they sanitized the dormitories of all migrant workers and also the malls and department stores in addition to various other public spaces including offices, restaurants, clubs etc. Various other measures like wearing a mask, social distancing, hand sanitization also were implemented. Here also an App Trace Together was introduced to track persons in quarantine. This App was later adopted and modified by the Australian Government and became a Covid 19 App.

A problem with migrant workers in Singapore was that many could not follow English or Mandarin. For them the Singapore government specifically introduced messages in Bengali (for the sizeable Bangladeshi workers) Hindi, Tagalong and Bahasa Indonesia. These measures seemed to have worked. While the Gulf countries saw an exodus of workers back to their home countries, Singapore did not see any such thing.

Singapore is famous for its vast number of restaurants, roadside eateries and hawker centers. Dining out was more or less the norm here and people had a huge choice here from the plush 5 star hotels to the one man or one woman stalls dishing out equally delicious food at much lesser prices. While social distancing was easy to enforce in the high end restaurants and 5 star hotels it became a challenge in the small eateries. However Singapore with its strict discipline and well known history of fines could do it very easily. Singapore also managed to successfully conduct general elections well into the pandemic.

South Korea which also had a massive spike in the initial days managed to control it fairly well with similar measures. In South Korea the initial spread was largely due to a church gathering. This was found out after eliciting a proper history and contact tracing. Finally a leading functionary of the church had to publicly apologize for the event and the subsequent spread.

In Malaysia the initial spread was due to persons returning from China. This was followed by an outbreak following a religious gathering by a group Tablighi Jamaat who organized a meeting in Petaling Jaya and that apparently led to further spread. Again measures like social distancing, wearing masks, sanitization helped control the infection.

Thailand was another country which was extremely successful as far as Corona is concerned. The reasons for that are not very clear but considering that it's a favorite travel destination across the world cases were much less here. Hot spots like Bangkok, Pattaya, Phuket, Koh Samui have almost become ghost towns with no tourists since March However the infection seems very well controlled.

Taiwan is another country in Asia that deserves mention. Even as mainland China and Hong Kong were getting flooded with cases Taiwan was left rather unscathed. Many attribute it to the safety norms and high rates of testing that were being done. They also attribute it to the considerable experience that the country had gained following the SARS pandemic. There was also a very able health minister Chen Suii Heng who is an epidemiologist by training. As soon as news of the Wuhan cases came in, the Taiwanese government started screening of all passengers coming from there. This was done much before WHO declared it a pandemic. They also prevented Wuhan residents in Taiwan from returning home. It also definitely helped that Taiwan was an island and the only way one could enter or exit was via air.

Vietnam, Cambodia Laos and Myanmar were other countries that lacked the glitz of their ASEAN neighbours but nevertheless they too did an admirable job. While Myanmar is largely controlled by the Army the others are not. However as compared to other countries tourist arrivals from Western countries was not that much even before the onset of Corona.

In Vietnam which is a one party country with no dissent, it was easier to enforce rules like quarantine. Also there were Short message services ent to everybody alerting them about the dos and don't during Corona.

In Cambodia on the other hand which is a relatively poor country things were similar. The country which had large number of garment factories quarantined as many as 15000 garment factory workers as part of its efforts to contain

Corona. Cambodia has a lot of unsanitary conditions including dust borne roads and a large chunk of people were already wearing masks even before Corona so the idea of wearing masks to remain protected was not a new thing for them.

Indonesia had a late start as far as Corona is concerned but unfortunately they continued to have rise in the number of cases. There are multiple causes for it. While most other countries imposed a lockdown fairly early Indonesia did it fairly late the reason being it would hurt the economy. This was a call that every nation had to take whether impose a lockdown or open everything and try to improve the economy. Another reason was the lack of enough testing centres in the beginning which lead to a number of cases. Another factor of Indonesia was its geography and the disparate different health system infrastructure in various areas

Sri Lanka was another country that had more than 1 wave of infections. After lockdown was introduced there and flights stopped, cases started plateauing bit. Thousand of Sri Lankans were working or settled abroad particularly in Canada, Australia UK, USA, Germany and New Zealand. There are also a huge number working in Gulf countries, Singapore, Malaysia and Maldives. Once flights resumed cases also started increasing.

One particular case was that of a patient referred to as patient number 206 actually a heroin addict who is said to have infected half the patients that Sri Lanka had till July. This happened basically because a navy team that went looking for him after he tested positive got involved in a scuffle in his village with other villagers. As a result of the melee several others including several navy personnel got infected. In spite of this however Sri Lanka managed to conduct a general elections. However in October the second wave came about and its spread was becoming a problem. One of those who tested positive worked in a garment factory in Minuwagonda and on further testing it was found that hundreds of cases had come from this point leading the authorities to label it as a cluster. Several deaths also occurred and many areas in and around Colombo are under curfew.

Yet another problem that was present in Sri Lanka was the disposal of dead bodies. As per Covid protocol bodies were to be cremated or buried at a depth of 12 feet or more. However Sri Lanka chose only to cremate the victims irrespective of religion. Other than Sri Lanka, China was the only other country to take such a step. This was done on the presumption that the Corona virus could spread through groundwater even if the victim was in a coffin. This led to several protests from the Muslim community as according to Islamic custom cremation was not permitted. The UN representative also said that there was nothing conclusive to say that it spread through groundwater. Maldives a friendly nation with ancient links to Sri Lanka chipped in saying that it is willing to bury all victims if the bodies are transported to Maldives. This led to even further acrimony saying that Sri Lankan Muslims should move to Maldives while they are alive so that they do not face issues like this. However this was eventually resolved after the huge outcry and negative publicity.

India with its vast population of 1380 millions had 10.3 million affected with deaths approximating 1.47 lakhs. Pakistan with its population of about 200 million had about 4.69 lakh cases with 9716 deaths while Bangladesh with a population of 166 million had about 5 lakh cases and about 7390 deaths. Overall it does appear that the Asian countries did better than Europe or USA if one looks at the number of cases or deaths per million population.

Another country that did remarkably well in actually flattening the curve and getting back fully to normal was New Zealand. Several factors worked in its favour.

Firstly it had population of only 50 million which was in matter of comparison half the population of the State of West Bengal. There was also a very low population density as compared to other countries Also it was an island or rather 3 Islands and the route of entry was only by air.

Also having a small population meant that the entire population could be tested. Another major factor there was that people there were basically law abiding and not given to dissent on government policies. Most important however was the role of popular Prime Minister Jacintha Arden and her leadership. She also managed to get elected for a second time during this pandemic.

In African countries the disease did make its entry in all countries but somehow didn't make much of an impact. As expected travellers to and from China from African countries were much less than say Europe or North America. Also perhaps lack of testing in the early days due to lack of testing centres may not have shown up the initial numbers as expected. But very few countries in Africa have had lockdown and most are back to business. In Nigeria one of the biggest African countries the number affected was less than a lakh. On the other hand South Africa which is one of the most affluent African countries the numbers are over 8 lakhs and the country is said to be experiencing a second wave. One of the reasons attributed to the second wave is the drinking parties that are currently on without maintaining Covid protocol like wearing of masks, social distancing, hand sanitation etc In Ethiopia the home country of the WHO chief Dr Tedros the number of Corona cases has actually seen a decline.

What explains this phenomenon in African countries. Apart from the fact of less foreign travel it is thought that cross immunity to other Corona viruses, experience in handling epidemics like HIV Ebola, outdoor living and a younger population also were contributory factors to this.

CHAPTER 13

What was the impact in India

While India had its first 3 cases in the last week of January and 1st week of February cases were rising elsewhere. As early as 12th February Rahul Gandhi de facto Congress chief tweeted quoting a Harvard journal that Corona is going to be serious issue and he is not sure if the Indian Government is fully prepared for that. At the point of the study the total number of cases in US had reached only 1500 but had obviously become serious enough to find mention in the Harvard Gazette. On March 4th Prime Minister Modi announced that he would not be taking part in the Holi festivities that was due to to be held in March. He also urged others to do so. On 19th March PM Modi addressed the nation 8 days after WHO declared Corona to be a pandemic and urged everyone to observe a Janta Curfew or peoples curfew on 22nd March. In his speech he mentioned the words Black out and Lockout and also lockdown. Having lived in the 70sin Kolkata or Calcutta as it was then called had memories of blackouts during the Bangladesh liberation war when lights were switched off at night with sirens wailing and also planes taking off.

Lock out again was another term which I learnt in Calcutta during the seventies and eighties which were the days of workers protests. There used to be strikes followed by some token attempts at agreement. If there was no agreement the owners had no option but to declare a lock out. Hundreds of establishments had lockouts those days many of which shut down permanently.

Coming back to PM Modi s address he urged everyone to be indoors from 7 am to 9pm on 22nd and at 9pm to clap or cheer for all the health workers and others involved in the fight against Corona. While this was widely welcomed by most people including film stars, sportspersons and others some of the Government critics criticized it vehemently saying Corona is not going to go away by such show of hands or claps. In effect it was a dummy run or a trial run for the lockdown that was to follow later. By now there was a feeling that something extreme is going to happen in India. Most colleges and educational institutions announced closure of their hostels and advised the students to return home. Similarly was the case for a few thousand migrant workers who managed to leave for their native places in time for Holi but did not return. By the last week of March many flights had already been canceled.

On 25th March Prime Minister Narendra Modi addressed the nation again and in a very bold move declared a 21 day lockdown that was to start from the 24th March midnight and end on the midnight of 14th th April. Prior to that Modi had video conferences with all chief ministers and apprised them of the situation Parliament which was supposed to carry on till April 3rd was adjourned sine die. While such a thing was always on the cards it was the suddenness that impacted many. For example many thought that sufficient time would be given say a matter of a few days or a week to get to places they wanted to reach. In many other cases people complained that they didn't have enough provision to last them 21 days. This announcement eventually took care of the Easter Holidays and also the various New years to follow in April including Baisakhi or Punjabi New Year or Poila Boisakh Bengali new year, Vishu Tamil. and Malayalam New year and Bihu the Assamese new year.

During the initial 21 days PM Modi after assessing the situation once again addressed the nation this time to extend the lockdown from 15th April to 4th May. Later on 2 further extensions were made from 4th May to 17th May and from 18th May to 31st May.

The first 21 days of the lockdown was the most effective. While only essential services were provided the police was out on the streets to enforce lockdown. But how were people expected to stay at home Someone in the Central Government decided to re telecast serials that were originally aired in the eighties and nineties in the Government TV channel Doordarshan. It may be remembered that those were the pre satellite television days and Commercial TV was in its infancy. However a number of hit mega serials including Mahabharat and Ramayan were made then. These were re telecast during the lockdown phase. And for many in younger generation who were born after the mid eighties it was indeed worth watching. Meanwhile the Government swing into action and there started a daily briefing of cases and guidelines While one expected the Health Minister Dr Harshvardhan himself an accomplished ENT surgeon to do the briefing in a daily basis it was left to a secretary in the Health department and officials of the ICMR to do so. While the Government like any other government across the world perhaps had no clear guidelines of its own due to the novelty of the disease and also lack of experience it had to borrow ideas from WHO and Centre for Disease Control CDC Atlanta and adopt them. Most of the guidelines were regarding social distancing norms, cough etiquette and wearing of masks While these were largely non controversial there was scope for finding faults with it.

To start with what were the masks supposed to be made of. Ideally it should have been N 95 masks that were initially used during the SARS pandemic.

However the problem was that it was costly at the start of lockdown forcing persons to wear cheaper surgical masks and cloth masks In later days however the production of N95 masks increased in the country and the prices also dropped. The second issue was the use of PPE or personal protective equipment. Again what were the components of this. Ideally it should have been a full Hazmat suit, Masks, gloves, face shields and gloves. This was not possible for a number of persons due to the cost Secondly a person wearing full PPE was not supposed to eat or drink or use the toilet something that effectively limited its use to about 6 to 8 hours. Another issue was the proper disposal of these PPE. While hospitals had their own bio waste disposal systems, the same was not true for the majority of individuals who used masks. While those who used surgical masks usually threw them away unscientifically or burnt them in the case of N95 masks was different. Many reused them after attempting to sterilize them. Apart from the quarantine guideline issued by the Government one of the guidelines was regarding deaths. As mentioned the guidelines the guidelines were taken from WHO and CDC who themselves had formulated this from events like the Ebola epidemic. In case of death the bodies were supposed to be cremated. If it was to be buried it was to be done at a depth of 10 meters Moreover no close relatives were allowed Instead it was done by local civic and health departments This was probably based on the Ebola epidemic where it was found that the practice of kissing the body led to a further rapid spread of the disease.

The other major issue was that of quarantine The disease was in an evolving phase in India and initially lockdown was for a period of 14 days initially in government designated centre with the person in quarantine paying for it And who were those who were to be quarantined. The government made some criteria which classified a person as low risk or high risk. He was considered high risk if he was not wearing PPE or was within 2 meters of the patient or shared the same toilet with him. Later on these guidelines were modified.

After the first lockdown states like Delhi Maharashtra and Tamil Nadu saw cases rising wrote to the Centre asking to increase the lockdown period which they initially extended till 5th May. Later that some restrictions began to be withdrawn and some states were declared as red zones in which the infection was high and restrictions were enforced. On the other hand in so called green states which had lesser cases restrictions were eased somewhat

So what did the general public do during the lockdown apart from watching television and being in social media through their smart phones.

Almost everybody worked from home. Online classes were held for students. This led to a lot of issues. In many parts of the country net connectivity was slow and power supply erratic. Many poor students did not have access to start phones or lap tops In many cases various social and political organizations chipped in and helped the poor students. In some cases post lockdown teachers actually went to the houses of these poor students to teach them.

Online teaching was not without its challenges. For the first time ever parents got a chance to actually see the classes of their children and that also gave them a chance to assess the teacher.

On the other hand some teachers who were not very tech savvy had to practice to come live before their students. While some schools insisted that their children actually wear uniform even during these classes the majority did not do so. Many teachers also had to make sure that there was no interference from other family members while taking classes something that was not very easy particularly if there are sick elders or small children in the house. Moreover the teacher had to look presentable and had to dress up formally even at home to avoid criticism.

It was a challenge though keeping kids at home after the online classes. These poor children used as they were to playing with their friends were cooped up in their houses. Luckily the smart phone came to their rescue and they do a lot of things in the virtual world.

Many others made use of this time to start or revive hobbies like cooking, singing dancing. A friend of mine a teacher to boot started showcasing her cooking skills on Facebook and You Tube and she has now got more than 2000 likes for her channels and You Tube has also started paying her for it. Others in groups started singing songs from various parts if the world and uploading them on You Tube. Modern technology had made this possible.

These hard lockdown days had many stories both funny, and heart-rending and sad. The early days of lockdown in Kerala for instance saw a few suicides of alcoholics who were not getting their quotas as liquor shops were closed. On the other hand one saw interesting and funny cases of violation of of lockdown restrictions. In one case a person had driven a long way with his friend trying to buy medicine for his pet cat. In another case a medical student was seen driving a car with the doctors emblem and on asking him which hospital or clinic he was attached to he replied that he was a medical student in Karnataka.

What was heart rending was the deaths. Quite some time ago I received news about a death of person I knew who died of a heart attack and not due to Corona. He expired at around 6 pm and his son was in Chennai and daughter in Bangalore. The person who informed me said that he will let me know the date of the funeral it was a non Covid death. The very next day I heard that the funeral was over by around 8pm as there was no way either the son or daughter could come. Several other cases like this are personally known to me. Some of these deaths that occurred after lockdown was lifted also had similar stories. A friend of mine who lost his mother in India could not come to India because commercial flights had not started from the country he was settled in. Another close friend who lost his father also could not come because it was simply not worth coming in the sense that he would have to be in quarantine for 2 weeks here as well as 2 weeks in the country he was.

During the period of lockdown all shops establishments, places of worship gyms malls etc were closed.

In the month of May lockdown restrictions were somewhat eased and the Government began the knotty problem of bringing back thousands of Indian citizens stranded abroad. Since no commercial flights were operating the Government bringing persons stranded abroad initially through its airline carrier Air India. Later private Airlines like Indigo, Go Air and chartered flights also joined this massive exercise was named Vande Bharat. In addition ships also brought in people from Maldives and Sri Lanka As expected countries with large Indian expatriate population got priority.

Among the vast Indian population stranded abroad were a huge number of persons who had gone to Gulf countries on a tourist visa with the intention of getting a job. The majority of them either stayed with their relatives or friends but there were no jobs in hand. Moreover they had run out of money too. Many others had come to join their children working there and were babysitting their grandchildren. There were several thousands across the world that had gone either for work or for sightseeing. In all these categories visa period was gradually ending. Howver keeping in mind the nature of the pandemic all countries extended their visas. While for senior citizens visiting their children and grandchildren it was alright since funds were not a problem, for a majority of the blue collar worker out on a visitors visa there was a shortage of money. Some had come with just enough money to make ends meet till the job offer came. However that did not materialize.

Here Indian expatriate organisations like Indian association and several others arranged for food and some money for them In case of those going on foreign tour and getting stuck things were different. While visas were extended and airlines agreed to refund charges there was little that the hotels could do. Consider this real life scenario a person and his wife due to depart to India on March 26th are stuck in Singapore as there are no flights and are due to check out that day. Obviously they had to stay till flights resume but how many hotels would allow them to extend their stay for free or even at reduced rates. While a few had the means to transfer money and stay on in the majority of cases they had to leave the hotel and go either to some friends place or seek the help of the embassy or the consulate. Many even took shelter in airports. To make matters worse there were reports of Indians dying abroad particularly in Gulf countries due to Corona.

Expectedly the first flights of the Vande Bharat flight were to Kerala which had the maximum number of expatriates working there. Those who wished to come had to register at the consulate there get a Corona negative test and then board the flight. They also had to download an App called Arogya Setu App. On arrival they would be taken to designated quarantine hotels where they would stay for 14 days. Initially airlines thought of keeping the middle seat in the aircraft vacant as part of social distancing but that would have increased the airfare as this was a flight for which the Indian government had pay the necessary parking and usage fees to the departing airport. Initially the testing before departure was not absolutely necessary but there was testing after 7 days after arrival in India. The initial passengers were selected based on their priorities for example a senior citizen or somebody with a lot of co morbidities needing treatment. It was indeed an interesting sight. When the first flight landed a minister was present at the hotel to receive them along with the district collector, local councilors.

And this trip was made from the airport in designated Ambulances with no family members present. It was quite a far cry from the early good old days when an NRI from the Gulf would be having a host of relatives and perhaps a good part of his village to receive him. His non family members would basically come to see if they could get some gifts from him or more importantly if he could arrange for a visa for them. After the arrivals of the first few flights came expectedly the number of cases went up leading the Chief Minister of Kerala to declare need that everyone coming here must get tested before coming here. There was a problem here as at that point in time the cost of getting a RTPCR was quite high and moreover one had to visit the hospital for getting tested something that itself was risky. The Congress led opposition in Kerala criticized the move saying that the Chief Minister was blocking the arrival of his own people by this step. Faced with this criticism the Government soft pedalled on the issue.

In between though several organization in the Gulf chipped in to pay the test charges for those who could not afford it. Several Indian organisations also arranged chartered flights to bring home the hundreds stranded since the demand for seats was rather high.

Meanwhile while Gulf countries remained the priority several thousands waiting in several other countries for which the Vande Bharat flights had not started. One of my former colleagues who was working in in international assignment in Mozambique was regularly calling me to find out if there was any update. His problem was multifold.

His assignment was over but he was in Mozambique in Africa which would have been very low on the Governments priority plan since the number of Indians were much less. Secondly when he first called me, his airport in Mozambique was closed. His normal travel plans was either Ethiopian airlines or via Kenya Airlines to Delhi with a change of flights at Dubai or Doha both of which were open but were risky since they were big hubs. Once Mozambique airport opened there seemed to be 2 choices open to him one was arriving in Mumbai and the other arriving at Kochi. In either case he would have to be quarantined While he was scared of getting quarantined in Mumbai because of the large number of cases he was interested in coming to Kochi and getting quarantined. But the question was would the Government allow it and considering his eventual destination was in Delhi. More importantly how was he going to get to Delhi after the quarantine in Kochi. He also toyed with the idea of taking a hired vehicle from Mumbai to Delhi in case he has to arrive in Mumbai. This was done in order to avoid boarding a plane with a lot of potential Corona cases After all these brainstorming sessions which he had with me he finally arrived in Mumbai and was put in paid quarantine there for 7 days tested between and then left for Delhi by flight to be in quarantine for next 7days.

Similarly another friend sent a message asking me about any news of Vande Bharat flights from Kazakhstan where her son was studying medicine Again like the African counties it was relatively low on the priority list and students from there got repatriated much later.

As arrivals increased it became increasingly evident that the system of paid quarantine would not work the way it was intended. For one, many of those arriving did not have the financial capacity to undergo hotel quarantine at their own expenses. So a decision was taken to quarantine them at home.

Similar was the case with several other persons coming from other parts of India.

Once lockdown was lifted there was another major problem the problem of persons wanting to return to their native places particularly the migrant labourers. While most institutions had closed down and most students had reached their homes this was not true of migrant workers in India road and rail services were yet to be restored. Many of the migrant labourers were on daily wages and productivity had come to a complete halt during the lockdown making their life miserable. Many of them were jobless with no money and wanted to go home but the question was how? Also they had to pay rent for the places they were staying in. While majority of landlords gave them a grace period for paying the rent some did not as the landlord himself was dependent on their money for survival. They also did not have money for day to day living including food. Here several organizations both political and non political chipped in giving free provisions to these poor labourees. In places like Kerala community kitchens were set up in almost all Panchayats. In the first week of May the Government announced running of trains in selected routes. Here the routes were based on the proportion of persons belonging to that are. For example Kerala had different trains proceeding to Patna,,Muzaffarpur, Bhagalpur and Katihar. These were special trains and did not have any stops encountered except for change of crew or engines. For boarding the trains one had to register at the concerned labour department which would be done usually through the contractor and then it would be confirmed after getting details of Adhaar card, mobile number Aroogya Setup App and other formalities. Initially a warm send off was given to those departing from these trains by officials from the railways and also those from the State government and elected representatives They were also given dry food and water to last them for their journey.

The were many stations that were not touched and since there was no public transport there was no way to go to their respective villages or towns even after alighting from a large station. For example a worker hailing from a village in say Jamalpur a not so busy station a small station would have to get off in Patna or Barauni or Bhagalpur to get to home. He would necessarily gave so travel 100 km to reach his home.

And there were plenty of social media messages that led to several incidents. In one such a Whats App forward said that special trains would be departing from Bandra, Mumbai leading to hundreds of migrant workers assembling there. There was a similar incident in Kottayam,Kerala also which said a special train would be departing for Kolkata from there leading to chaotic scenes there also. Meanwhile parents of students studying in coaching institutes in Kota,Rajasthan (a town famous for its coaching centres for engineering) managed to put pressure on some state Governments to bring back their children studying there. This obviously led one to the question as to why migrant workers were not given the same facility. This was also a time for political parties to pander to their constituents. As early as on the 4th h day of lockdown thousands of migrant workers headed for the interstate bus terminals in Delhi in an effort to reach Uttar Pradesh. While both the UP government and the Delhi Government had arranged for about 1000 buses each it was simply not enough. Many missed the buses and started walking to their respective villages. Some of them were picked by Good Samaritans on essential duty who ferried them for part of the way while others just collapsed out of sheer exhaustion. One day it was found that quite a few had fallen asleep on a rail track and had been killed. It was indeed extremely tragic.

Another callous instance was that of trains ending in wrong destinations. This was rather surprising because unlike normal situations where there are hundreds of trains this time there were very few trains all across the country. Also in today's modern high tech world one had devices like smart phones and Apps like Google maps It still remains a mystery how such things happened. Admittedly the announcement of lockdown as expected was sudden and nobody in India had any previous idea of this and whatever information one had was through the counties like China which enforced a lockdown however in only some parts of the country. Clearly our bureaucracy and its implementing officials were not fully prepared for this particularly with an extremely large migrant population. Meanwhile the Finance Mnistry set in a set of measures to help the economy. Money was disbursed to the states and while loans were not written off a moratorium of a few months was given. However this led to some protests saying that while the moratorium was fine the individuals still had to pay the equated monthly instalments or EMIs something which was becoming difficult with loss of income and in many cases loss of jobs.

CHAPTER 14

In India different states adopted different methods to deal with a rapidly evolving disease.

Delhi was one of the states that was hit very badly in the early stage of the pandemic many cases were then linked to a s meeting organized by a religious sect Tablighi Jamaat that also had meetings in Pakistan and Malaysia and were also partly responsible for early outbreaks there.

In Delhi it was found that many members who participated in this meeting were foreign nationals and quite a few had overstayed. Many of these persons also spread out to other states like Maharashtra and Tamil Nadu. In a short span Delhi, Maharashtra and Tamil Nadu became the leaders in numbers along with Gujarat. In Delhi just a few months ago elections had been held and the Aam Aadmi Party led By Arvind Kejriwal had won elections. Simultaneously there was also large protests going in against the Citizenship Amendment act which had been passed in

Parliament but had resulted in a lot of protests. While the protests started as early as December they now seemed focused in an area of Delhi called Shaheen Bagh which had become the focal point for all opposition politicians. Although it took a bit of time the protestor left the venue once lockdown was announced. Soon the number of cases in Delhi many prominent persons including politicians and bureaucrats started testing positive. While Delhi had a number of Central and state owned hospitals it was also home to many of the seriously ill from adjoining states like Uttar Pradesh and Haryana. There were also high tech hospitals both in Delhi and adjoining NOIDA and Gurgaon. And that where the first roadblock started. It was obvious that not all patients would get admitted into Government hospitals but it was found that many persons got admitted into private hospitals. Private hospitals on their part raised their fees astronomically literally fleecing the public. But actually that was not entirely true. For example if a doctor or a nurse had to be on 6 hour duty before Corona there was no extra charge apart from the bed charges, medicines and doctors fees. But here there was also the cost of PPE which at the minimum was about 1000 Rupees including Hazmat suit, Goggles, gloves, masks, shield. In a 24 hour shift it would be 4 such sets for a doctor and nurse or a total of 8 for both together. This led to a total of Rs 8000 extra per day for this alone which was obviously added on to the patients bill. There was also the cost of RTPCR tests which was about Rs 3000 This inflated bill led to huge outcries and a cap had to be made for the exorbitant bed charges. In the meanwhile health care workers were getting affected and a few also died in Delhi.

Later the Government decided that not all who have tested positive need to get admitted as gradually beds were getting full. Those with mild symptoms could be treated at home giving them good nutrition in the form of vitamins. In some cases antibiotics like azithromycin, and steam inhalation were also given. There were however many patients in intensive care units and many needed ventilator support as well.

Meanwhile volunteers of Aam Aadmi Party started house to house visits checking oxygen saturation of individuals something that was innovative and did have a good feel about it. After the initial surge in April and May there appeared a decline in the numbers which some said was due to low levels of testing. It was later rectified and tests rates started going up again. However the test positivity rate had come down to about 3 percent after the Diwali festive season.

The disease however claimed the life of India's former President Pranab Mukherjee who just before getting admitted to hospital tweeted that he had tested positive. Others who were affected included the Home Minister Amit Shah and the Vice President M Venkiah Nadu. While the Vice president was in home isolation the home minister had to be admitted to hospital.

Maharashtra was one of the worst hit states for Corona and continues to be so. Again while initially outbreak was said to both due to the religious gathering of Tablighi Jamaat whose members had spread all over the country there were also others who were effected. The most badly hit were Mumbai and Pune. Mumbai was the country's financial capital and was home to some of India' richest persons. It was also home to Bollywood Indian film industry. One of the earliest patients from Mumbai to get affected was veteran superstar Amitabh Bachhan who tweeted that he had tested with his family and actress wife Jaya Bachchan son Abhishek daughter in law Aishwarya Rai Bachhan and granddaughter had to be admitted into a private hospital while his wife and daughter in-law were discharged fast after testing negative Amitabh and his son Abhishek had to spend a few stressful days and nights in the hospital. Here was Amitabh an actor in his 70s who had suffered from Tuberculosis and hepatitis in the past and survived a near fatal injury earlier in his carrier who came out successful in his battle against Corona.

One feature of both Mumbai and to a lesser extent Pune was the presence of housing societies in multi storeyed buildings. These were established perhaps in the 60s and 70s and started spreading all over. There existed a camaraderie among the residents and the society usually framed its rules. Once the outbreak was announced these societies swung into action. Maids and other household helps were not allowed to enter. The security staff were given hand held thermometers and would record the temperature of any resident going out or coming in and if there was a increase in the temperature that would be informed to the concerned person for taking necessary action. Apart from maids and household helps, other entrants like milk delivery boys, newspaper boys etc were prevented from coming. Each occupant tried to ensure that he or she was safe as also his or her neighbours. But not everybody lived in such a, multistoried building. One of the first places to witness an outbreak was at Dharavi which was Asia's largest slum s pread over an area of just 2.1 sq km it was home to a million people making it one of the most densely populated areas in the world.

Here was the underbelly of Mumbai the average Mumbaikar who eked out a living somehow and lived in unpretentious surroundings unlike those of film stars or the societies. An outbreak here was proving to be a challenge because of the sheer density of the population and the surroundings which were far from congenial to healthy living. However the Brihan Mumbai Municipal Corporation or Greater Mumbai Corporation and the government health staff went on an overdrive going for massive testing with the result that in a months time Dharavi had stopped reporting cases although the number of tests remained high. In December there was zero case reported from Dharavi. In Maharashtra again the story of hospitals getting full, patients being overcharged and health workers falling victims to infection was there just like Delhi. It had become so serious that the Government actually called for doctors from other states to come and help. Many doctors and nurses did go to help for a short period. During lockdown everything was closed and even after lockdown train services which was the main mode of transport for thousands was stopped. However a few suburban trains did run and their services were only for essential Government staff who had to show their identification at that point of entry. Quite early into the pandemic organizers of Ganesh Chaturthi the biggest festival of Maharashtra spread over 10 days decided that this year there would be no festivities and instead the money collected for the same would be distributed among the poor.

Gujarat also had a early rise in cases. While Gujarat does have a large NRI population with plenty of Gujaratis having relatives in USA and UK it was unclear as to where the initial spurt of cases came from. Some persons and sections of the media attribute it to the visit of President Donald Trump to Gujarat on 24th February for the Namaste Trump that was organized there. At this point of time USA had a fairly large number of cases which Trump was downplaying in his characteristics style. The World Health Organisation had not yet declared it a pandemic either and number of cases in India was very less. If one follows the epidemiology which says that the incubation period is between 7-14 days it means that some persons could have caught the infection and because it had minimal symptoms they never tested Also they could have passed on the disease to someone else in another 7-14 days by which time WHO had declared a pandemic. However lockdown was declared much later in March 26th. About 1 to 1.25 lakh persons attended the event and apart from PM Modi and a few other dignitaries like the Chief Minister of Gujarat Mr Rupani or the Governor nobody could even come very close to Donald Trump. However part of the entourage including Secret Service personnel as part of standard operating protocol had to necessarily arrive before Trump at all the places before him. It was never thought at that time that the disease could occur to anybody other than someone with a recent travel history to China. Later however the number of cases declined in Gujarat.

Tamil Nadu had a similar incidence of high number of cases. It was again it was initially attributed to returnees from the religious event conducted by the Tablighi Jamaat in Delhi. Later on returnees from abroad and other states contributed to it. One focal point was the wholesale market at Koyambemedu which was one of the places responsible for massive spread of the disease. The market had to be closed more than one occasion for a few days.

However increased testing in the initial phases helped in controlling the spread of infection to a large extent. The Tamil Nadu government has traditionally been one that dishes out populist ideas be it the Mid-Day meal program or much later establishment of Amma canteens which supplied food at extremely low rates. This was no exception. Here the government provided multivitamins, Zinc and also advised persons to take a particular solution developed by the Siddha department of Indian system of medicine part of the AYUSH which stood for Ayurveda Siddhartha and Homeopathy. Apparently some of this did work and Tamil Nadu s cases came down.

Orissa was another state that was interesting from another point of another point of view. Every year the famous temple town of Puri hosts the annual Rath Yathra or Chariot car festival usually attended by lakhs who pull the chariots of the presiding deity Lord Jagannath his consort Subhadra and his brother Balaam. But how was one to do this during Covid times? Following a public interest petition in the Supreme Court the Chief Justice initially stayed the Rath Yathra as it poses a great risk to the spread of Corona. However public sentiment was in favour of holding the Rath Yathra. Accordingly the state government appealed in court for holding the Rath Yathra, even in a symbolic way. Finally the Supreme Court withdrew its stay and permitted the Rath Yathra with several curbs in place. Only 500 persons including the temple priests and others were permitted. Moreover all of them had to undergo a RTPCR test and prove negative before participating. All Covid protocol was to be maintained. No vehicles from outside Puri were allowed here and Puri itself was to be put under curfew. Details of those participating were to be noted and shared with the health department. The Court also observed that Rath Yathra was responsible for spread of plague and cholera in earlier centuries and observed it would be difficult to follow up on those participating. During this screening for Corona one senior priest of the Temple was found to be positive. However there was no marked rise in the number of cases here.

In adjoining Andhra Pradesh things were different. The famous temple of Tirumala in Tirupati district which is one of the richest in the country and has staff of 22500 had opened its doors in June and by July it had had 700 cases including some priests. One former head priest too succumbed to the disease. One state that kept itself free from Corona for a very long time was Sikkim. This was bit surprising because Kalimpong in adjoining West Bengal had a number of cases in the beginning However Sikkim tightened its borders not allowing in any tourists. The first case occurred in late May however and cases have been rising ever since then.

The only place that has not witnessed a single case in India has been the Lakshadweep Islands which is a Union Territory and only accessible by flights or by ships. With both of them yet to resume services it was but natural that cases here would be close to zero or zero.

CHAPTER 15

West Bengal had a different picture The first case was that of a student the son of a very senior bureaucrat who had returned from UK. This case raised eyebrows because this student had gone partying and only got tested when he developed symptoms and was admitted in Infection diseases hospital Beliaghata This incident occurred on 8th March.

On 18th March the first death occurred of an elderly man who had not been abroad but according to some reports his son had been to Italy recently and had returned from there. Just after lockdown was declared there came unconfirmed reports about deaths from Bengal in social media. There were viral clips about bodies being buried in a hurry under police protection. The opposition parties in West Bengal were quick to accuse the Government of West Bengal of a cover up. India is a federal country with several states many of whom are at loggerheads with Centre's ruling party the Bharatiya Janata Party or the BJP. What was worrying was the apparent number of deaths as mentioned in the social media. Now the Chief Minister of West Bengal Mamata Banerji set up several committees for Corona. It was however the formation and action of a death audit committee that raised eyebrows. This was because if a person tested positive for Corona and died the papers or documents would be sent to this committee that would determine whether it was due to Corona or co morbidities like diabetes, cancer, hypertension etc. In effect would bring down the official Corona deaths a lot. More importantly this led to considerable delay in getting the death certificate since the approval of this committee was needed. There was another knotty problem. In case of a Corona death the body would have to be cremated or buried as per Corona norms while for others it was just a normal procedure. While it was true that co morbidities were also contributing to deaths the primary cause was indeed Corona.

Critics of this gave an interesting analogy. Suppose a patient with hypertension or diabetes gets run over and killed in a road traffic accident would one consider it as an accident or a death due to hypertension. In the wake of this a Central team was sent to West Bengal on a fact finding mission. In conformation with the political climate there was initially little or no cooperation from the State Government who stuck to their stand.

Eventually though the State Government had to comply with the Centre and classify all deaths with tests positive being that due to Corona irrespective of whether there were co morbidities.

The first of several deaths of health care workers also occurred in West Bengal. One of those who died due to Corona early on was a assistant Director of the State Health department a senior doctor. This expectedly lead to more fears particularly among the medical fraternity. By then cases had begun to rise in numbers and some hospitals were declared Corona hospitals. There were also designated Corona care places like stadiums and other places. Soon after declaring some hospitals as Corona hospitals came another issue. There were many non Corona patients taking regular treatment at some of these state run hospitals. These were basically persons with chronic disease requiring chemotherapy (cancer patients) dialysis for kidney patients and repeated blood transfusions for patients suffering from thalassemia and anemia and leukemia. Where were they supposed to go? In case of some of the hospitals with multiple buildings it was possible to make one building or part of it and exclusive Corona care unit but in many cases it was just not possible since the infrastructure of the wards was set up in such a way that different floors had different departments. As cases increased so did the number of containment zones and in the initial days there was a lot of resentment against the containment zones. While some residents felt that their area was given a bad name by labeling it a containment zone, others resented the fact that they could not get-out of the barricades guarded as it was by the police. Chief Minister Mamata Banerji had to personally visit some containment zones to pacify the persons living there. In most of these areas the residents were daily wage earners and their sole source of income was cut off. However the police and other Corporation officials stepped in to see that their daily requirements were taken care of. Similarly Kolkata had a high percentage of senior citizens who were staying alone as their children were away mostly abroad or in some other state. While Covid restrictions meant that they could not go out it also meant that they would be greatly affected. In many places household helps like maids had been forbidden and that was indeed another not so trifling matter to be taken care of. However much earlier the Kolkata police had a helpline for senior citizens staying alone and many used this facility to get things done. There were also the locality boys who chipped in to help their uncles and aunties For elders while this was alright what was more difficult was the finance and the medical care. While quite a few did become tech savvy and were able to use Epayments using Apps the majority had to depend on hard cash for getting things done. While there were thousands of pensioners the problem was to go to the bank to get withdrawn for daily use. In a few cases where the senior citizen was quite friendly with the manager of the bank often a bank staff would come and hand over the cash.

Another problem was medical consultation for diseases other than Corona. Senior citizens due to their very age were more prone to non communicable diseases and would often go to doctors for monthly or fortnightly check ups. Corona regulations meant that it was not possible. However most doctors and hospitals offered teleconsultation facilities. In many cases the doctors would recommend continuing the same medicine for a month or more. Emergencies of course was something different.

A major problem here was for the existing post graduate trainees and the house surgeons or interns. Most of them were on Corona duty and this meant that for quite a long period of time they would see only Corona cases and nothing else. This meant that a house surgeon posted in say orthopedics or dermatology or a Post graduate in those subjects would necessarily see less of the cases he is supposed to see as a junior doctor. Moreover his Corona duty apart from being risky was also causing severe anxiety and stress.

By this time Chief Minister Mamata Banerji who was rather skeptical of Corona began to realize the problem and started enforcing rules.

Lockdown meant also that transport stopped. This included the oldest Metro Railway in the country the Kolkata metro as also the local trains and buses. The Kolkata metro is considered the lifeline of Kolkata much like Mumbai suburban trains and even long after restrictions were lifted it continued to be closed. Similarly local trains also continue to be closed while local buses in Kolkata resumed service soon after lockdown was lifted And since metro railway services were stopped there was a maddening rush in the buses throwing all social distancing norms to the wind.

Yes masks were there but that was about it. Passengers were in packed buses like a tin of sardines as a result a majority of commuters who normally use metro services began to use the already strained buses.

Bizarrely though flower markets and sweet shops were kept open. While the Bengalis known for having a sweet tooth the fact that many couldn't live without them was surprising. Moreover with places of worship being closed what on earthly use was the flowers for. A friend quipped you are buying the flowers for your own funeral and the sweets are also part of it.

At around the same time the Kolkata corporation started a house to house campaign asking for persons with any history of fever, cough, headache and getting them tested. This was done in almost all wards.

By March there appeared another issue that impacted the Corona issue. That was the arrival of Super Cyclone Amphan. Warnings were given much earlier and many relief camps were set up in anticipation. There was a basic contradiction because Corona protocol demanded social distancing while relief camps meant that persons would be in close confines of each other. Although the duration of Amphan was less its impact was huge and it mainly affected the South Bengal districts of Kolkata, Howrah, South 24 Parganas and Northern Parganas. In rural areas of South Bengal impact was the worst several houses were destroyed electric poles were uprooted and roads damaged. The Centre had already sent in National Disaster Relief Force NDRF teams before the cyclone and sent in more after the impact. Prime

Minister Modi on a request by Chief Minister Mamata Banerji himself came just 2 days after the cyclone hit and sanctioned an interim relief of Rs 10000 crores. In Kolkata the impact was different. Hundreds of electric poles and tress were filled by the cyclones. The main issue was with the trees falling on electric lines and the electric poles getting uprooted there was no electricity in the majority of places. Most people were on the streets protesting or giving soundbites to local channel. It was not without any reason Without electricity it was impossible to pump water to the first floor and above. This in effect meant an absence of both water and power two out of 3 of the famous combination of Bijl, Sadak or Pani or electricity, roads and water the USP for any political party. However the power was restored in a few days after the NDRF teams did tremendous work in removing the debris caused by cyclone Amphan.

One of the pastimes of the average Calcuttan precisely Bengali was the daily marketing and Adda, or informal get together. While the arrival of Supermarkets have changed the lifestyles of many, there are several others who can't live without going to say Gariahat or Manicktala or Newmarket to get their fish and fresh vegetables. As one of my worthy Bengali friends said nothing like going to such a place feeling the fish and then haggling over the price before buying it. This also came to a stop during the lockdown period and for quite some time later Another pastime was that of Adda which was basically a chat usually in a small restaurant or better still in the open air sitting on a parapet that is colloquially known as the rock. While the origins of this are not known it basically attracts men of all age groups. While those unemployed used to be the majority there also used to be large numbers of employed persons who would join in before heading home or come here after freshening up at home It would be usually over tea and cigarettes with a vegetable or egg or chicken chop or fish fry or cutlet thrown in for good measure Topics of discussion would range from simple neighbourhood gossip to more higher things like politics, sports, cinema the arts. Again this camc to a stop in Calcutta.

The timing of the lockdown extending as it was over the Easter holidays and the Bengali new year had severe economic impact on trade. While Easter per se did not ever effect trade much there was the Chaitra month year end sale that was severely impacted Chaitra sale the Bengali month that ends just before the start of the Bengali New Year which is usually on 14th or 15th April. This sale which is a year ending sale is one of the two biggest sales occurring in Kolkata the other one being the Durga Puja sales later in September or October. Shopkeepers give huge discounts and in normal situations it would be almost impossible to shop at leisure in places like Gariahat one the traditional shopping areas.in Kolkata. Moreover the impact of cyclone Amphan added to the woes particularly of the small time trader.

Once lockdown restrictions were lifted trains started plying but these trains basically carried migrant workers. Although the Railway ministry ran the trains the permission of the state in which the destination was located was needed. Bengal did not give permission for trains carrying migrants returning to Bengal for fear that the disease may spread a fear that was not totally unfounded was only later after opposition parties started protesting that she finally relented. As far as quarantine were concerned it was clear that quarantine in designated hotels would not be an option for migrant labourers from other states and the majority quarantined themselves at home. After Amphan expectedly the number of daily cases rose in Bengal crossing 3000 per day. A little later with further unlocking flights also started coming in Apart from the few Vande Bharat international flights there were also domestic flights. However Chief Minister Mamata Banerjee did not give permission for flights coming in from cities with high number of cases like Mumbai, Delhi, Chennai etc matter a few weeks though this order was withdrawn.

However more was in store for West Bengal. The Government declared a weekly 2 day lockdown.

The purpose of this was not known but was ostensibly to prevent persons from moving about freely on all days. Cynics, asked whether Corona virus was aware of the lockdown dates. What was more bizarre was that there was no fixed day. One week it would be Monday and Friday as the lockdown days while another week the days would be Tuesday and Saturday. Till now very few people even those in the close circle of the Chief Minister have not been able to understand the relevance of the days. The last of these days was just before Viswakarma Puja which marks the apart of the festive season in West Bengal. While Viswakarma is said to be creator of the universe and his puja is usually confined to factories offices there is puja done of all machines including cars, bikes buses and there are also Pandals with idols of Viswakarma. This festival is also marked by kite flying plus a celebration with good non vegetarian food and liquor. After Viswakarma puja there is usually Mahalaya the start of the Durga puja festival and is it marks the descent of Goddess Durga from her heavenly abode to be on earth for10 days culminating in Vijaya Dasamii the day she vanquished the Half Buffalo half Asur or demon Mahisasur. This time though, the Bengal almanac brought about a gap of 1 month from Mahalaya to Vijaya Dasami. Meanwhile Maharashtra with it spiralling cases had decided not to have Ganesh Chaturthi celebrations another festival that lasts for a long time. In the absence of clear instructions most Durga Puja organizers started getting ready for Bengal's largest festival that spread for over 5 days Many had made grandiose plans with various themes for pandals. As part of the preparations a meeting had been convened and organizers were asked to maintain Covid protocol. This initially meant that all pandals would have 4 sides open in contrast to earlier use 1 or 2 sides open.

But how was one going to stop the thousands of people from going there. It was not clear. On the one hand there was tradition to be maintained. On the other there was Covid protocol to be maintained. One of Kolkata most famous pandals at Santosh Mitra Square also called Lebutola colloquially was the first to announce that they would not allow anyone to visit the Pandal. While some Pandals are usually located at parks the majority are not and one to go through narrow lanes and barricaded queues to reach the Pandal.

The pandal at Santosh Mitra Square was one such. Pandal. During normal times a Puja like this would attract footfalls of 50000 per day. Meanwhile Gujarat banned its famous Dandiya Garba dances which were done every night during Navratri or the 9 nights that form part of Durga Puja or Dussehra. Meanwhile other states like UP and Bihar, Delhi also put curbs on festivities.

Meanwhile the opening up of the shops and the arrival of pujas meant a near return to normalcy. There are a few shops in Kolkata which attract customers during Puja season and a famous leather showroom situated in Lindsay Street is one of them. Even in the best of times it is very crowded not to say of Puja shopping. Soon viral clips of frenzied shopping without at this shop flooded WhatsApp and other social media. Meanwhile Pujas arrived and as is customary the Chief Minister went on a puja inauguration spree. It is a convention now that the bigger pujas get inaugurated by the Chief Minister or other political heavyweights. Some of them also get inaugurated by film stars Planning for pujas start months before and lakhs of money come through sponsorships apart from individual house to house subscriptions. There are also several competitions for various categories for including best Idol, Best Pandal, Best Theme,

Best lighting, Best décor, Best safety measures and so on. While Chief Minister Mamata Banerji inaugurated the puja pandals physically in many cases taking maintaining protocol the same day saw huge crowds at one of the big Pujas. Sreebhumi which had made its pandal based on the famous Kedarnath temple and which the Chief Minister had inaugurated just a few hours ago. Meanwhile so viral footage of this crowd also flooded social media. The very next day the High Court admitted a petition asking for safety measures in view of the crowds. While another counter petition was filed by some persons representing certain puja organisers the court decided that not more than 50 persons would be allowed in a small pandal and not more than 100 in a large pandal. This included also the priests the drummers or *dhakis* and the organizers themselves. The Court also said that failure to implement this would lead to serious consequence. Many pujas arranged for live telecast of their Anjali (an offering to the goddess). The high Court order also said that there would be no Sindur Khela a ceremony in which the married women gather and apply Sindur or vermillion on the idol on the day of Vijaya Dasani the last day before the idols are being taken for immersion. Also the practice of giving traditional hugs or Kolakolli as it was called was stopped.

In short it was a win win situation both for the chief minister her party and government and also the others who wanted tradition to continue The sponsors too were happy as their money also did not go down the drain completely.

The courts came to the rescue again during Diwali and Kali puja festivities While the number of Kali puja pandals are much more than the Durga Pujas the chances of people visiting in hordes was much less.

CHAPTER 16

Kerala which is one of the most developed states in India and scores heavily on social economic and health indicators was the first state to get Corona cases in India In recent years Kerala which has had a good record in communicable disease control had its record spoilt slightly by the high rise of Dengue cases there in 2017.

In 2018 2 major health related events occurred.

The first was the arrival of hitherto unknown disease Nipah affecting 2 of the Northern districts Calicut where it made its first arrival and adjoining Malapuram district. While bats were thought to be the source of infection there were contradictory reports in the presence if virus among bats. This disease which spread really fast also caused several deaths. It remained unclear however how the virus came to Kerala. The disease was first described in Malaysia in the nineties and pigs were the reservoirs of infection and once pigs were culled the infection was over in Malaysia. After that the disease appeared with regular frequency in some districts in Bangladesh where toddy tapping was a main source of income for the villagers Farmers would keep pots to catch the toddy in the night but bats would feed on them and also in fruits. People would get infected after consuming either the toddy or other fruits consumed by bats. In West Bengal the disease was observed in 2 districts of West Bengal that border Bangladesh i.e Siliguri in Darjeeling District and Nadia While in Siliguri the diagnosis was made much later after the outbreak the outbreak at Nadia also involved health care workers as well as close family members. Here too toddy tapping was identified as one of the factors. However in Kerala the index case had no history of toddy tapping. Also bats were not known to have such a large flight range from west Bengal to Kerala about 2500 km. Also while bats including fruit bats were present everywhere cases where only reported from Kerala. What was the apparent reason?

Was it that the other states were not doing testing Or was it something else. Anyway Nipah was finally declared under Control by June 2020. This short period of 1 month saw 19 confirmed cases with 17 deaths including that of the brave nurse Lini Puthuserry who contracted it from the first patient who was under her care at EMS

Cooperative hospital Perambra. WHO and the Central and state Governments acknowledged her valour and she received the Florence Nightingale award in India posthumously. All over the world Kerala received praise for the effective way in which the outbreak of Nipah was controlled in such a short time although with 17 deaths out of 19 infected. Much of the success of this goes to health minister K K Shailaja Teacher who is not a doctor but is a science graduate and had a clear concept about what was going on Just prior to this. I had the opportunity to attend a meeting addressed by her and the health secretary outlining the States preparations for the monsoon season. The focus at that time was in dengue as the previous year had several cases and Nipah was unheard of. I was actually a bit surprised at her knowledge and understanding of the subject and her receptiveness to ideas. During the Nipah outbreak Shailaja Teacher led from the front visiting the victims houses and also Kozhikode medical college and other private hospitals where people were under observation. By the first week of June the diseases disappeared from Kerala as mysteriously as it appeared.

There was also a hit Malayalam film called Virus based on the Nipah outbreak and Kerala's handling of it It subsequently dubbed in other languages. There was another solitary case the next year too i.e 2019 but that was it.

Just as Kerala and the rest of India was amazed at Kerala fighting an epidemic there came another piece of bad news. In August Kerala saw the biggest flood in the century and all districts except Kasaragod the northernmost district were severely affected. While heavy rains was the cause what aggravated it was the almost simultaneous release of water from all major dams. Hundreds of houses were damaged and hundreds died. The National Disaster relief teams or NDRF teams were pressed into service very early into the rains. In a rare gesture the Chief Minister Pinarayi Vijayan and the leader of the opposition Ramesh Chennithala undertook a joint aerial survey. This was followed the very next day by a visit from the then Union Home Minister Rajasthan Singh who apart from doing an aerial survey also visited some of the relief camps set up. Prime Minister Modi himself came on 17th and did an aerial survey but could not complete what he had planned to do because of inclement weather. Thousands were stranded in their flooded houses while many had shifted to relief camps The Army,Navy and Airforce too was called in to render help. After the rains stopped came there was the massive task of rehabilitation. This was one area in which almost the entire Kerala chipped in shedding their political or religious affiliation. The first part of this was obviously to arrange for food and medical aid at the relief camps Many socio cultural, political and religious organizations helped with relief and rehabilitation. Meanwhile financial aid came in from all quarters Apart from the Central Governments fund and the Chief Minister' Relief fund funds started coming in from other states. Many other states sent their medical teams also to help in the medical and relief activities. Once things were somewhat stabilized in the relief camps there came the problem of shifting the persons back. In most cases while water levels had come down many houses where damaged and needed repairs. Local masons and plumbers were roped in for minor repairs. More important was the onerous task of cleaning the houses quite a few of which had begun to get occupied by reptiles. Here again locals armed with cleaning equipment including gloves, masks, bucketd disinfecting solutions stepped in and ensured that the houses were made habitable.

The aftermath of any such flood is the presence of epidemics. This was more likely in a place like Kerala which had dengue, leptospirosis or Weil's disease and diarhoeal diseases as major infective diseases. Fortunately everyone was given tablets of Doxycycline which resulted in very few cases of Leptospirosis. Also the intense cleaning activity after the flood made the houses look spanky again and there was little space for mosquito breeding sites thereby reducing the chances of mosquito borne diseases like Dengue. Moreover after the flood there was more awareness and more hand hygiene practices were adopted. By around November 2018 Kerala had become almost normal barring some damaged houses.

With such a robust and efficient government including the health department in place it was a surprise when the first case of Corona in India was announced as being from Kerala. This was a medical student from Thrissur who was studying in Wuhan, China and managed to catch a train to Kumming just before lockdown was announced. From Kumming she flew to Kolkata and after an over night stay in Kolkata she flew to Kochi and then came to her home district. By then instructions had gone to screen passengers coming from China and this student tested herself at the local hospital and when the result came it turned out to be positive She was then shifted to Thrissur Government Medical college In another couple of days 2 more cases both medical students also tested positive for Corona and were also admitted in Government medical colleges At that time it was thought that this would be affecting only people from China and these students though infected with the virus appeared to be healthy By this time apart from China places like Iran, Italy, South Korea also began to show increases and the Government of India started screening persons coming from here also. Here however there was a catch. There was no direct flight from Iran or South Korea or Italy to Kerala and the concerned passenger could get away with concealing his travel itinerary particularly if he had changed flights at Dubai or Doha. Things were apparently alright till March 8th when a group of persons all hailing from Pathanamthitta district contracted the the virus in leading an elderly couple What happened was that that a middle aged couple with a son who was settled in Italy decided to come to India but for some reason they hid the fact that they came from abroad. It was only after their neighbor's were admitted to hospital with symptoms and a detailed history was taken was it known that they had mingled with the family who had come from Italy. In the process quite a few got infected including their aged parents who were well into their eighties. This led the normally affable Health Minister to burst out during a press conference almost blaming them for spreading the infection. She and the Chief

Minister also proposed stern action if such a thing were to get repeated. By this time the well oiled health department got into work and started the first ever contact tracing. This was done by a dedicated team over telephone and involved asking the person where all he visited and who all he met in the past 7 days before he was diagnosed. This gave a list of his primary contacts and then these primary contacts were in turn contacted to find out their list of of contacts who were the secondary contacts. While primary contacts had more potential to get infected a database was also created of th secondary contacts. This list obviously depended on the places he visited abd the number of people. Meanwhile cases also began to get reported from other parts of Kerala.

A group of foreigners who were supposed to stay confined to their hotel in Munnar were tested for Corona but due to a procedural snag they left the hotel before the results came and headed straight for Kochi Airport to catch the flights back home at the last minute The national lockdown had not started as yet. They were literally prevented from boarding the flight as the manager of the resort informed the police and the tests were also positive and they were immediately taken to Government medical colleges for treatment. Those in the same group but who were negative were also admitted watching for symptoms. Again the whole process of contact tracing was done. Soon stories of new cases came from all over. There was for example a tourist from Italy who was apparently a regular at the seaside town of Varkala near Thiruvanthapuram. This gentleman went around almost half the town, attended DJ parties and also danced at a temple festival and had taken several selfies with the locals and posted it on social media. This gentleman also became missing and it took some time to track him. This person's primary contacts went into more than a thousand.

Similar was a case of another passenger from Gulf hailing from Kasargode the northernmost district who got off at Calicut Airport and then travelled first by car to Calicut city and then by train to Kasargod. He seemed to be a very sociable kind of person as he attended a couple of weddings a funeral witnessed a local football tournament, went for prayers although 2 different mosques also took selfies with at least 2 elected representatives Members of legislative Assemblies. It was common enough for returning NRIs non resident Indians in Kerala to visit their relatives and take part in social functions. However in this particular case also the contact list went into thousands. There was also another case of a small time politician who was based in Idukki but travelled across several districts meeting several persons including ministers and other officials at Thiruvanthapuram the state capital. It was soon becoming increasingly difficult to do contact tracing. By this time though lockdown had been declared and cases in Kerala were slowly rising but not as fast as neighboring Tamil Nadu or Karnataka. Soon people started to praise Kerala for its efficient handling if the situation as compared to that states like Tamil Nadu Karnataka Maharashtra and the health minister Shailaja Teacher received praise all around for the splendid work that Kerala was doing Apart from BBC, Reuters, Washington Post WHO and several other international media organisations interviewed her. In one of these interviews she stressed on strategic testing. The aim she said was to keep the test postivity rate at about 2 percent. At this point of time, states Maharahtra, Tamil Nadu and Karnataka all had test positivity rates above 7 and in some cases above 10 percent Critics said that it was due to Kerala doing fewer tests among the population. Unless more tests were done it was impossible to get more postives they contended. In the month of April the average number of tests done per day was below 1000 while other states had gone into 10000 and 20000 ranges. It was thought that a possible shortage of testing kits could have led to this low number of tests. Soon in the month of May the testing was ramped up and the number of cases also went up. By the beginning of May the Vande Bharat missions started and as expected so did the number of cases. Meanwhile the chief Minister of started a daily live telecast of Corona updates. This was telecast at 6 pm every evening Indian Standard time and soon become a hit particularly among the non resident Malayalis This was followed by a small question answer session. In no other state in India was any Chief Minister giving such a briefing regularly.

It was becoming increasingly evident that not everybody could afford the paid quarantine at hotels selected by the Government. The Government then decided to allow home quarantine which was quite the natural thing to do. Many of those in quarantine did not have attached bathrooms and therefore several other institutions like college hostels and other such campuses were taken for the purpose. Soon Government hospitals began to run out of space and private hospitals were also asked to keep a part of their beds ready for Corona care. Government also declared that treatment expenses for Corona patients in private hospitals would be borne by the state government. Another feature that was noticed that many of those who tested positive were asymptomatic and could be easily managed at home if they did not fall in the high risk group which meant people with co morbidities like diabetes, hypertension, chronic obstructive pulmonary disease COPD, cardiac patients etc Keeping this in mind first-line treatment centres or FLTC were set up where relatively healthy persons who tested positive were kept and observed by a medical team. If symptoms increased they were shifted to the nearest hospital.

The Government had issued orders for the elders to remain at their homes and not venture out. Kerala had an aging population with majority not having their children staying with them. For these persons volunteers from various departments including health department gave them all the help they need. There was also another issue here In case a young person from the household is positive then the elders were taken to specific Reverse Quarantine Centres where they stayed with similar persons in similar situations However latter concept of reverse quarantine centres did not meet with much success as many elders were reluctant to leave the confines of their familiar surroundings. There was also the risk of overcrowding at these reverse quarantine centres which would have defeated the very purpose of this whole exercise. By this time the number of cases had increased manifold and it was not just due to returnees from abroad or other states.

In the month of May once lockdown restrictions were eased somewhat, road traffic resumed. Trains and domestic flights were yet to start though. Soon the number of vehicles coming in from Maharahtra, Tamil Nadu and Karnataka started coming in and so also the number of cases. At that particular time in May Maharashtra Tamil Nadu and Karnataka had many more cases than Kerala. Along with these infected passengers frontline workers like police who were checking records and noting addresses also started getting affected. Also health workers started getting affected in fairly large numbers clusters started forming particularly in areas which had camps or dormitories like police camps, CRPF camps (Central Reserve Police Force) BSF (Border Security Force). Also there were cases among other closed community residents like those at old age home, nuns in convents and priests in seminaries. Both returnees from other states and returnees from abroad contributed to the number of cases. By this time quite a few deaths also occurred. One such death was a person who suffered a head injury when a coconut fell on his head. He was taken to hospital and while testing for Covid they found he was positive.

In June however the tests went up and the number of postive cases also increased and for the first time ever the Chief Minister Pinarayi Vijayan announced that community spread may have started. Once lockdown restrictions had been lifted educational institutions, places of worship, gyms, cinema theatres and malls continued to remained closed all other standalone shops and supermarkets opened. And to make up for the lull during the lockdown there began a mad rush particularly to well known departmental stores and textile Emporia. And sure enough some if these textile shops had to be closed down temporarily after it was found that staff developed Corona. By June end while the number of foreign returnees and domestic arrivals among the Corona cases remained the same there was a fairly large group in which the source of infection was not known.

In July there was another incident that had an indirect impact on Corona. Following a tip off the customs intercepted a package addressed to the UAE consul General in Thiruvanthapuram. On questioning it was found that a lady who had worked earlier in the UAE consulate and was presently working in a Government of Kerala undertaking was the main person behind the racket. It was also learnt that the lady was appointed through recommendations from higher ups including the Chief Minister's personal private secretary a bureaucrat. Soon the case was taken up by the Centre and multiple Govt agencies including Customs, Enforcement directorate and Ministry of Home Affairs. Once the Chief Minister's private secretary was called in for questioning the opposition lost n time in protesting. Both the Opposition UDF United Democratic front and the BJP lost no time in getting into the streets and organizing massive protests in spite of Covid protocol regulations in place. While the lady and the bureaucrats were taken into custody the opposition bayed for more blood and hit the streets. Many cases were charged but it was fast becoming a daily drama. The Chief Minister and Health minister warned that cases will go up after this agitation which it did. The health minister went a step further and said that daily numbers could cross 10000 something which did happen in reality. After the request from the Government to call off the agitation the opposition was clearly on the backfoot. Whatever support they would be getting from the people as a result of the war against corruption would be nullified by the loss of groundswell due to the rising number of cases. And the LDF had already absolved itself of anything and squarely put the blame on the opposition for their reckless agitation which was risking the lives of thousands. Faced with this scenario the opposition had no other option but to cancel it mass agitation. Cases started to be reported from markets including fish markets which resulted in fish markets being closed temporarily This in turn resulted in people not buying fish for a few days.

There were several stories regarding Corona victims. During the initial days persons in quarantine tried to run away This included even an officer of the Indian Administrative Services who managed to reach his home state even as he was supposed to be in quarantine. He was issued a show cause noticed and subsequently suspended. No doubt it was a very trying experience being in quarantine even though there were several calls by support staff including consultant psychologists and medico social workers.

Quite a few admitted to hospital with Corona tried to attempt suicide and a few died also It was the fear of a dreadful disease and the possibility of death that forced them.

Covid protocol for deaths involved either creating the bodies or buying them below 12 feet. Here was one problem. Some districts like Alleppey for example were on the coast and the water levels caused problems in burials In another case the body of a victim who was a Christian was not allowed initially to be be cremated in the Hindu crematorium by locals. It was resolved only when the district administration intervened. Again the Church was supposed to oppose cremation as compared to burial as it was against the tenets of Christianity. Here again the family of victim wanted the cremation of the body to take place as per the Government protocol in the local church to which the church authorities refused initially Finally the administration had to intervene. Subsequently however bodies of Christians who died due to Corona were actually cremated in church cemeteries.

While the opposition stopped their agitation on the streets another factor came that influenced the Corona outbreak. This was Onam the main festival of Kerala. While official Onam celebrations were banned what was not banned was the Onam sales. For a consumer state like Kerala to miss out on its sales firstly during the Easter and Vishu was bad enough but that was common to all states in India Again another major sales was during Ramzan and Eid both of which were impacted by Corona. So the only imminent thing was Onam shopping. This would help the ravaged Kerala economy which had little to cheer for in an otherwise extremely gloomy years. And sure enough the state was full of buyers who were totally oblivious to Covid protocol. By this time by-election to a few assembly constituencies was due This was necessitated by the death of existing MLAs. Simultaneously the terms of the local self governing bodies including Panchayats, Municipalities and Corporations were also due. The Election commission postponed the by elections for assemblies but curiously gave the go ahead for local body elections in Kerala. The term of local bodies in West Bengal too had ended earlier but the Government and the state election commission were in no mood to conduct it for whatever reason. Just some time ago Bihar had successfully conducted the assembly elections which was preceded by huge rallies all wearing masks but generally not abiding to the rest of the protocol. However Bihar had far less cases than other states. More recently in Hyderabad elections were held to the Greater Hyderabad municipal corporation. However the elections in Hyderabad saw a low turnout with polling percentages below 50 percent. Evidently the majority of voters in Hyderabad decided that its better to be safe than be sorry later.

In Kerala once the polls were announced it was back to business for all political fronts. While the ruling LDF was trying to prove that it had done its best with several welfare schemes that benefited the common man the opposition UDF and BJP was trying to wrest power from LDF and the main plank was corruption. The question was how to get the voters to the polling booths. Election officials announced that persons with Corona would be allowed to vote either as a postal vote or physically after all the votes in the booth had been cast. The problem was for persons in containment zones and those in quarantine. Also there were questions about senior citizens who were told to stay at home as part of Corona protocol but were courted by political parties for votes. And local elections are by and large based on personal popularity and accessibility of the candidates and micro level local issues rather than state or national politics Also the margins of victory in many of these seats are often wafer thin sometimes even in single figures. So every vote counted. The voting percentage was quite high about 77 percent so. While protocol was maintained in terms of social distancing, wearing of masks, hand sanitization and barring children from booths the presence of elders did raise a lot of eyebrows. The impact of the high voter turnout during these elections is yet to be known as the elections were over only in the second week of December. This was followed by another frenzy of shopping this time for Christmas. Again the impact of this will only known in the time to come.

In the month of November was the traditional Sabarimala pilgrimage that started from mod November lasting for 41 days. This was restricted to men and also women who were less than 10 years and above 50 years or basically those women outside the reproductive age. This was based in an age old tradition that women of that age should not take part as the presiding deity Sabarimala Ayyapan or Dharma Sastha was a confirmed bachelor. This temple was in the midst of controversy 2 years ago when the Government based on a court ruling tried to open the temple for all leading to a confrontation between traditionalists and modernists who argued from the gender equality plank. The matter is still in the Supreme Court of India for a final judgement but at present the status quo is being maintained meaning women of reproductive age are not permitted. The temple itself is located atop a mountain amidst a forest nestled at the Western Ghats and has to be covered in foot for about 3 km quite an arduous climb. A large majority of pilgrims were from other states like Tamil Nadu, Karnataka and Andhra Pradesh. There were also pilgrims from Kerala who also would take part a in this after observation of vows for a period of

41 days This included celibacy, taking vegetarian food and abstaining from vices like alcohol and cigarettes. For convenience the days used to be shortened. It was also a common sight in pre Corona days to have local Ayyapa pujas in most areas or temple and often at homes after which the pilgrims would head to Sabarimala. This was in normal times a big source of revenue for the Government. Starting with travel operators, taxis, hundreds of road side stalls selling food and drinks and stalls selling puja related items it served as source of indirect and direct money for hundreds if not thousands.

However with Covid restrictions in place this year was different. Firstly train services were not restored fully. Secondly pilgrims coming by air or by road had to prove that that they were Covid negative This year again there were no local pujas. The number of local pilgrims almost become nil in spite of the Government permitting a maximum of 5000 pilgrims per day Altogether it was a different Sabarimala that one saw.

Another major temple was Guruvayur in Thrissur District which is managed by the Guruvayur Devaswom The Devaswom has a monthly expenditure of Rs 150 crores but since the lockdown there has been hardly any income. Two events that added to the income were Marriages and rice feeding weaning ceremonies of babies s at 6 months called Choroonu in Malayalam. While feeding ceremonies were completely banned as there were children who were prevented from going there as part of Covid protocol restrictions the case of marriages was different. Although solemnnized in Guruvayur these were done outside the temple premises on platforms called Kalyan mandaps. Here marriages were allowed restricting the total number of persons on the Mandapam including the photographers. Also there were restrictions on the number of persons who attended the sumptous lunch that followed. Guruvayur was conducting its annual Ulsavam or festival when lockdown was announced. Another important event was Vishu or Kerala New Year which occurred during lockdown. After lockdown restrictions were released came Ashtami Rohini or the birthday celebrations of Lord Krishna the presiding deity of Guruvayur. This too was a low key affair restricted by Covid protocol This was followed by the Ekadasi celebrations which did see a lot of participation but there were curbs on the entry of persons into the temple. In December however it was found that quite a few employees including some priests contracted the infection and entry was banned completely A random check of employees of the Devaswom revealed that more than 500 had contracted the disease. The area around the temple too became a containment zone.

So looking at it from a broad perspective how did Kerala fare in Corona control? At one point of time it was hailed as the state which had flattened the curve Today it is he state with the maximum number if active case. What exactly were the possible causes?

The first possible cause could be the self confidence that was present once the first few cases came. This stemmed largely from Keralas' widely acclaimed health system. There was as also the fact that Kerala had handled the much more fatal Nipah and the floods that followed. However this confidence later turned into over confidence which proved to a major reason for the failure. Another reason in Kerala was the fatigue factor For a state which had the first 3 cases as early as January the health system was getting battle weary. There seemed to be no weapon in the arsenal save the vaccine which was yet to come People were continuing to do things like contact tracing and psychological counseling for months together.

The second one was the self patting by the powers that be as soon as Kerala met with some initial success when the cases were low and it was doing much better than its neighbouring states. The health minister of Kerala Smt Shailaja Teacher was the role model and she was being praised nationally and internationally. Not unexpectedly the opposition started criticizing it saying it was due to excellent public relations by the left and its friends in the media. There were health ministers in every state they said and nobody boasted of the achievement of these health ministers though in many cases the number of cases was much less than that in Kerala. For example not all media persons knew the names of the health ministers of Tamil Nadu, Delhi and other states which also brought down the numbers. A very senior Congress leader from Kerala made a rather disparaging statement against the Health Minister Shailaja Teacher and later had to apologize for this statement. However rather than fight Corona unitedly as in other states the parties were feuding among themselves. Once when the Union Health minister Harshvardhan said that there was a spike in the number of cases after Onam a state government employee junior in the hierarchy but prominent on channel discussions and social media made a post in social media criticizing the Union minister saying he was playing politics. He had to finally remove the post after a backlash on social media and the intervention of the Kerala Health Ministers. In no other perhaps was there so much politics over Corona. In Bengal for instance the BJP and CPM were against the Trinamul Congress which was the ruling party but there was not much criticism after the initial days. Similar was the situation in Maharadhtra, Delhi, Tamil Nadu, Karnataka an other states.

Another major cause for the rise in cases was the frequent change in guidelines and the adaptation of Central guidelines to the state.

Take for instance the guidelines regarding high risk and low risk cases. Anybody who was within 6 feet distance or without PPE was considered as high risk. What constituted PPE was not fully clear. After March 24th everybody or nearly everybody wore a mask and therefore would bd in the low risk category. This categorization was also based on telephonic contact in which one could not make out the body language of the person. Even if somebody was not wearing a mask at that point time he would say that he was actually wearing a mask. It was like a policeman asking a person suspected of robbery whether he committed the crime or was present at the spot. Speaking in hindsight it would have been better to keep all contacts in quarantine for a few days rather than classify them into low risk and high risk. It was probably the low risk population who were acting as silent carrier. Another example would be if a nurse working in an ICU who is wearing PPE and us hence classified as low risk and is asymptomatic. Being low risk and asymptomatic mean that she would not need testing although she could be harboring the virus. She could be a latent or silent carrier much like Typhoid Mary a cook who infected persons on both sides of the Atlantic.

Another circular by the Central Government said that in case of reinfection there would no retesting of the individual since RTPCR is known to remain positive for over a month while Rapid Antigen test would give false negatives. Some persons interpreted this to mean that negative test was not mandatory for persons rejoining work. This was something very dangerous for health care worker who could be returning to work with the virus and instead of stopping the chain would actually be continuing.

Another aspect has been the behavior of the people. While in the initial days people were scared of the disease once lockdown restrictions were lifted people began to feel free and less scared. They felt that it was just like any other flu and while one may get hospitalized it was usually the very elderly i.e those over 70 and those who had co morbidities who had real risk of dying. Along with this realization came the careless behaviour, going for shopping without sanitising hands, going for parties and much more.

Also although from time to time the government talked of strict measures in case of any violation of protocol hardly any cases were charged.

In the end though Kerala's figures are not very encouraging. For a population of about 35 million cases it has over 7 lakh cases including more than 60000 active cases and over 3000 deaths. It is indeed true that most deaths occurred in elderly persons and many of the cases occurred in persons coming from other states or countries The figure of some other states are very telling.

In Maharashtra for example which is the worst hit state the total population is 114 million with 1.9 million affected and has 49,124 deaths.

In Uttar Pradesh the total population is about 204 million and about 6.6 lakhs are affected with 2941 deaths.

In Bihar with a population of about 128 million roughly the same as that of Maharashtra the number of cases is 2.49 lakhs with deaths at around 1377.

Evidently having the same population doesn't necessarily mean the numbers are likely to be same or similar as in the case of Maharashtra and Bihar.

Chapter 15

What was the effect of lockdown on the world and economy in general What was its effect in India.

Across the world the economy collapsed. The travel and tourism industry remained most affected. Hundreds of hotels across the world were forced to either lay off staff or close down indefinitely permanently. Vacations became a thing of the past. Fine dining outside was reduced to takeaways. The likes of food delivery apps like Swiggy, Uber eats, Zomato etc took a big leap in their business.

In many cases the restaurants closed because they couldn't get customers In several other cases the chef or the other staff couldn't rejoin for work due to travel restrictions.

Worse was the hotel and airline industry. For any hotel to be successful it had to have at least 30 to 50 percent occupancy and this was simply not happening. While some governments did give some incentives to support the hotelier many found it to be too little.

As far as airlines goes the case was worse. It was impossible to keep the middle seat vacant as suggested by many as a measure for social distancing. This was because that would have entailed a higher cost to the passenger per flight something which would have deterred the passenger from flying and that in turn would have put another nail in the coffin of these airlines.

Consider a international flight with say 30 rows each of 9 passengers with a total of270seats capacity.

Keeping the middle seat vacant would mean that that there could be only 6seats per row or 180 passengers. Assuming that each ticket costed 100 dollars the airline was getting an income of 27000 dollars from with the new regulation it would result in an income of only 18000 dollars and for getting to that figure of 27000 dollars each passenger would have to pay more.

Many airlines tried a lot of things to tide over it. One was just boarding the aircraft with security check and boarding pass ready but the plane would be stationary. Even food was served in the flight. Some airlines went a step further and organized flights to nowhere which meant that the flight would take off but land at the same place obviously at an increased cost.

Major airports like Changi Airport Singapore,Dubai Doha etc bore the brunt of these as they were the ones with heaviest traffic.

The fear of travel is going to be there for quite some time. Gone is the planned vacation with family in some exotic place. While some countries like Maldives have opened up in a big way (it has virtually no other option as its only industry is the tourism industry) others like Thailand and UAE are doing it cautiously.

In Thailand for example a person who wants to go for even a short visit has to book for a 14 day stay in Government designated quarantine hotel. Moreover he must show enough funds through bank statements for the stay of 14 days and also must have adequate medical insurance quite a tall order for many. Indeed a far cry from the earlier visa in arrival when all one need was proof of booking in any hotel and minimum funds.

Another major change was the cancellation of meetings and conferences the world over. With travel restrictions in place and hotels not opening, conferences and meetings went into virtual mode with the Zoom platform being the one being used the most. While it did result in a lot of savings for the organizers it was nothing like the real thing where one could interact physically with others

More importantly for conference regulars it also meant the loss of a stress free period to chill out and the absence of good food at the conference venue.

Another big casualty of Corona has been the educational sector. Every single class had to be done in virtual mode In a vast country like India with erratic net and power connectivity in some places it really became a challenge to organize this. There were several others who did not have a laptop or smart phone either In many case though various organisations and individuals helped out these poor students by giving out free laptops, smart phones etc In a few reported case there were reports of persons going up the roof or climbing small trees to get net connectivity. This also happened in Malaysia and other South east Asian counties in in addition to the Indian subcontinent Online teaching apparently alright but what about online examinations. It was as not possible to asses the person for the simple reason that one did not know if the student was using unfair means like asking his family members or copying from texts. This continues to be a great deterrent. The case of Medicine was even more difficult. While theory classes were done online it proved impossible to do practical since that involved direct interaction with a patient something that could not be done during the pandemic. Giving a simulation or case study is a good idea but not something like the real thing. This is indeed a significant matter in the course of medical education mandates that every person should pass the practical separately.

In case of competitive exams though things were slightly better. Examinations for medical and engineering exams were held using Corona protocol in offline mode because the numbers were large and it was not possible to have so many centres with online facilities. In exams to other universities though like law and others it was online and many exams gave the candidate the benefit of sitting in ones home and giving the exam in other exams specialized centres with wifi connectivity were used as the venue. This again led to some technical glitches for many who were not used to this and instead were also more familiar with the pen and pencil mode. Obviously people with better net connectivity could possibly do better in these.

One of the biggest casualties in this great pandemic has been the entertainment industry particularly the movie industry. With projects worth millions in the pipeline there was no shooting during lockdown and even after lockdown was lifted there were no shooting. This was because of travel restrictions by air and also mandatory testing for all such. Also interstate travel had not really picked up making outdoor shooting difficult. There was of course no question of shooting in a foreign country However many filmstars were stuck in foreign lands where they had gone for shooting. One such was Malayalam film star Prithviraj who had gone for the shooting of a film Adujeeitham based on a novel by noted Malayalam writer Benyamin. This novel and the film dealt with the not so comfortable life of a migrant worker from Kerala It was directed by noted film director Blessy and the shooting was in Jordan and initially permission to shoot was given for 2 weeks in the historic Wadi Rum desert in Jordan in March. Soon after that flights in and out of Jordan were stopped and a few support local staff had to quarantine themselves. The entire crew of 58 including the director and actor had to stay in Jordan for a total of 73 days returning only towards the end of May. This was a real harrowing experience for the entire team On the other hand with cinema theaters yet to resume screening it was bad days indeed The film industry of old had already been dealt a blow much earlier with the advent cable TV and CDs and DVD. To make things worse people stopped coming to old fashioned theaters. Many of these theaters occupying prime space shut shop and instead came shopping complexes Many of these malls were multiplexes meaning there were multiple halls screening multiple films Although ticket rates were higher than that of a normal stand alone theatre it was a different experience altogether. A family of four would in average spend about 2000 to 3000 here These were also extremely popular with the younger generation. However with the lockdown and its aftermath these too suffered heavy losses.

In some places there were attempts to open theaters with full covid protocol in place but there was hardly any audience and the theaters remained shut.

Another sector that was shut was saloons and beauty parlors. During lockdown they were completely shut and during this period some persons tried cutting and styling their hair at home often based on YouTube videos. Some persons even called the local barber home Often help of family members were taken for this. Once lockdown restrictions were lifted a few gradually returned to saloons and beauty parlours and the person cutting the hair or styling it was supposed to maintain covid protocol as far as possible. No less a person than Indian Prime Minister Narendra Modi went on to grow his hair and beard over 8 months.

Chapter 16

One of the key areas that was hit by Corona was the field of sports. Japan which was due to host the Olympics first postponed it and finally decided to conduct in 2021. Almost all other sports with spectators and involving close contact were canceled in the wake of the pandemic. India is one of the most cricket crazy nations in the world and one of the regular events in its calendar was the Indian Premier League or IPL which was in its 13th year. Here there were only 8 teams but they would play against each other in multiple centres followed by a 2 semifinals and finals. World cricket has evolved a lot from the early days when there was only test cricket spread over 5 days in which there could be result or it could be draw. In a few instances there were ties too But that was when people had more time. Later on came the one day cricket internationals in which teams played against each other usually playing 60 overs per side initially but now the number of overs per side has been reduced to 50 overs. This format gave India its famous World Cup victory in 1984. Later on even this format was modified into Twenty Twenty where each team could bat or bowl a maximum of 20 overs. This effectively meant that each side would effectively bat for about 100 minutes or so and the match itself would be over in less than 4 hours. For the purists it was not very inspiring but for those who wanted quick action this was it Either hit out or get out would be the motto. This was played both among cricketing nations and also in various leagues where teams would be formed with members coaches, doctor, fitness trainer etc. In addition these matches would be streamed live on Channels and each advertising slot would command a huge amount from various countries However these players would be auctioned by various franchisees and top players or very promising players would automatically be auctioned at higher prices. The franchisee on the other hand would make their money either through advertising their teams through television or selling merchandise. Various companies would be also associated with franchisees adding to their income. There would also be a huge support staff starting from manager to coach to bowling coach batting to trainers and fitness coaches In short this raked in huge amount of money for the board of Control for cricket in India or BCCI. This year though Corona changed the plans of IPL. As all the players had been bought, advertising rights as well telecast rights had been brought what was to be done? The tournament which was played initially from March to May was postponed. A little later the BCCI toyed with the idea of having the players play in empty stadiums since the number of cases had gone up although the lockdown had been lifted. Finally it was decided to shift the tournament to UAE which had far less cases than in India. The UAE had also hosted a n earlier edition of IPL in 2014 in normal non Corona times when the tournament had to be shifted out due the General elections.

Around the same NBA hosted Basketball under a bio bubble in Orlando, Florida, USA The bio bubble basically meant that all safety precautions were taken regarding Corona virus. The reason for choosing the UAE were many Apart from the number of cases the stadiums at Abudhabi, Sharjah and Dubai were closer to each other and could be easily reached by road in a very short time unlike India where travelling to different venues would entail flights in some cases a change of flights and long waits in airport. This was simply increasing the risk manifold. Also UAE had prior experience in hosting the IPL and also had a robust health system.

However playing in this bio bubble was not going to be easy. Each person had to undergo 5 tests for Corona While 2 of the tests them had to be done before reaching UAE. the other 3 were done within 1 week of landing. Every member of the squad had to undergo this including the officials.

In addition they also were quarantined for 14 days and on the 5th day of every week everyone was tested all over again. Apart from testing what was important was the segregation of players who were not allowed to meet each other in hotel rooms or lobbies. They also had to quarantined for14 days after arrival in their respective countries.

This edition of IPL played out over 2 months in front of empty stadiums proved to be tremendous hit with very few persons falling ill due to virus. One must complement the excellent work done by the organizers particularly Saurav Ganguly President of Board of Control of Cricket in India and also the UAE authorities for successfully conducting the tournament in the midst of Corona.

CHAPTER 17

One of the key factors has been the role of testing Test, test more was the underlying message by the WHO.

The question is what tests? While RTPCR continues to be the gold standard there have been issues in its utilisation in India. It is free in the Government sector while costing about 2700 in the private labs. The problem with the Government sector was that due to the vast number of cases the results would take more than a day. In some cases the person would not get a copy of the result because only positive cases were given results. In contrast Rapid Antigen test is much cheaper costing about Rs 700 only and gives results in a few hours The problem with Rapid Antigen test is that it has a high number of false negatives. This effectively means that a possible subclinical case though RAT negative could be actually be having the virus and could potentially spread it to someone else. In case of RTPCR the problem was that the person could move about freely till the results came thus leading to potential spread of the disease. Generally all cases for admission in a hospital were subjected to RTPCR if the patient was going for a planned surgery or Rapid Antigen testing if it was an emergency admission.

Many countries across the world set up testing kiosks In India also several testing kiosks were set up.

Here came another question. Who were the persons doing the tests.

In pre Covid times throat swabs were done basically for detecting streptococcal infections in rheumatic fever a disease that is rather uncommon now. Now most laboratory technicians were not doing this throat swab both due to relative rarity of this disease and also more specialized tests. However all the testing is done for Covid is done by medical and paramedical staff who ideally should have been trained in this technique. Unfortunately due to the huge numbers and no hands on training thanks to Covid restrictions quite a few may not be adequately trained. So is it possible that some cases may be missed due to faulty technique like the swab not reaching the correct place due to the gag reflex present in all of us or because the concerned investigator for obvious reasons wants to do it very fast? The answer to this is not known at present. Again a few persons have questioned the naso pharyngeal swab saying that in case of a dry nose it may be difficult to get the sample Also if the person has been taking any nasal drops like Otrivion or Nasivion containg Metazolinr or oxymetazoline the chances are that the virus may not be detected. This again is debatable.

Coming back to RTPCR versus RAT testing the daily figures of testing do look impressive What not mentioned is the number of RTPCR and number of repeat cases. Repeat cases are those that were positive earlier and have become negative now. To give an example a state has done say 60000 tests out of which 6000 are positive give a test positivity rate of 10 percent. But if there are say 6000 tests that are repeat it would mean that there are 54000 new tests that are done. Keeping the same figures of 6000 positive with 54000 tests the test positivity rate goes above 10 percent. If the repeats are 10000 then the test positivity rate goes much higher at 12 percent. Again if one looks at the percentage of RTPCR tests among the total tests most states have the percentage of RTPCR hovering at below 25ercent. Very recently Delhi has had another wave and instructions are out to increase the percentage of RTPCR to over 50 percent.

CHAPTER 18

What exactly has been the role the World Health Organization in this whole pandemic. The WHO did not exactly cover itself in glory during the pandemic soon as the first cases came some time in December last year the warning bells should have been sounded. Even much later when the province of Wuhan in China declared a pandemic WHO remained rather guarded in its response labeling it as a case of maximum risk but stopped calling it a pandemic. It was only on March 11 that it was declared as a pandemic. Could things have been different had an emergency been declared earlier After all just a few years ago we had the SARS pandemic and more recently outbreaks of Ebola.

It's difficult to answer this in hindsight but before that one should understand the functioning of the WHO.

It is for all practical purposes an organisation funded by various Governments. Per se WHO has no funds of its own. Elections to the coveted chair of the director General are also made on political grounds. One also has to take into account world politics particularly that involving China from where the virus is said to have originated from and the USA which is one of the biggest donors to WHO and which has also got the maximum number of cases. There is also the trade war between US and China. The present chief of WHO Dr Tedros hails from Ethiopia and is a former minister there but he is not a qualified MBBS doctor However he has considerable experience in the health sector which is why he stood for elections and subsequently won. Also WHO does not have an army of doctors or consultants across the world in adequate numbers though there are region specific and country specific offices. There are also consultants and surveillance medical officers for specified diseases like tuberculosis, polio, measles, and neglected tropical diseases.

Coming back to Corona while the first case actually came to attention in December 2019 the sequencing of the virus came only in January At that point of time the strict Chinese regime while releasing the details of the virus did not cooperate fully with WHO With a strict media control by the Chinese Government and an obvious language problem any information was hard to get by. It was only after the Hubei lockdown that pressure mounted on WHO to declare it as a pandemic To be fair to WHO they took more than a month to declare it a pandemic mainly because of economic reasons. After all declaring a epidemic as a pandemic affecting several countries has its severe repercussions on trade and travel which would hurt the global economy. By March 11th almost all countries had started reporting cases This delay led to a diplomatic war of words between China and the rest of the world mainly USA. Many reports said that China was the cause of the disease and its spread while a few suggested that the virus itself was man made in a laboratory in China.

After declaring it a pandemic there started a daily briefing by WHO n its headquarters which apart from om giving general directives also lauded individual countries on their work.

In India like possibly in other countries too the work of WHo has been minimal India does have a country office and New Delhi is the headquarters of the South East Asia region. As a former Surveillance Medical Officer of WHO for its polio program I would like to share a few experiences of the past where WHO and WHO SEARO South east regional office had moved in. During the aftermath of Tsunami my colleagues based in South India actually went out and helped in the relief and rehabilitation.

In 2008 I had the good fortune of being part of a training for Emerging and Reemerging diseases preparation for a pandemic This was done jointly for short service assignment holders both from polio and from TB and this was done just before SARS.

In 2010 while I was posted in Pakur, Jharkhand we had our first case of Polio in July that year and an entire team of approximately 12 of my colleagues came to help me from other parts of India. Similar was the case in Sahibgunge in Jharkhand and also in Murshidabad in West Bengal. Thanks to these reinforcements we managed to knock out the virus of polio from India and while the last case of polio in India was reported from Howrah, West Bengal 8 out of the total of 42 cases of India in 2010 was from my district of posting Pakur. Obviously team work did help.

After 2011 some of my former colleagues in WHO were sent to Nigeria on more than one occasion and successfully contained the virus there also

More dangerously there was yet another mission by WHO India in controlling Ebola in Sierra Leone a mission that was extremely hazardous.

In contrast the effort by WHO this time has been rather lacklustre possibly because of the criticism of WHO by USA and by other countries. The Epidemic act was brought about health remained a state subject an it was left to states to find out their own resources to combat it. Most states chose their own state governments health department. To be fair the honorable Union Health Minister of India did have a teleconference with WHO staff but nothing really tangible came out of it Admittedly WHO doesn't have enough field staff for a pandemic like this since quite a few offices have closed and downsizing has occurred.

In Kerala for example while the SMO was involved in the initial few cases it soon became an avalanche which WHO could not handle. In Bihar there was a house to house survey done by health workers in the beginning of the pandemic which the WHO SMO Surveiilance medical officer had to monitor, but that was just about it.

So how could WHO have brought about any change if at all in handling of epidemic. For a start we have a fairly good epidemiological case investigation for Acute flaccid paralysis surveillance or AFP surveillance which contains details of the person including symptoms, travel history history of health seeking behavior, date of examination laboratory result etc. This had a unique number with the first 3 letters being that of the country them the state then the district then the serial number. A simple modification of that could have been used for entering the data which was foolproof. This data for polio and entered in EPI Info a statistical software package early ensured there was little scope for duplication in the data.

Another huge data bank which is there at least in states like Bihar,Jharkhand and possibly Uttar Pradesh also is the microplan which contains the names and addresses of every single household Use of this initial stages of the epidemic would have correctly identified clustering of cases and potential hot spots.

In Bihar there was a house to house activity basically done by health workers to find out persons with symptoms of Corona. This activity was monitored by WHO field staff. While the correctness of interviewing persons and the genuiness of the data collected thus can be questioned it does appear that Bihar has done very well in containing the virus. Not only that Bihar also successfully conducted assembly elections with massive rallies during campaigning without adhering much to Covid norms. Yet there was no great surge as expected.

There was no surge in Bihar also after the Chath Pooja which is the biggest festival in Bihar which is dedicated to the Sun God although thousands thronged the river ghats where offering and Puja is done to the Sun God during sunrise and sunset.

In Jharkhand also there was a house to house campaign this time by Accredited social health activists or ASHA workers who also did a lot of awareness campaigns including wall writings with messages about the signs and symptoms of Corona.

Overall though the involvement of WHO left much more to be desired. There are reasons for this one of which is the WHO role globally. In the case of polio we had a very effective vaccine and as it was an eradication program funds were in plenty. Although the program took a lot of time to yield results in the end there was success.

CHAPTER 19

One feature about this pandemic is the relative lack of knowledge regarding the disease Modern medicine or allopathy as some would name it has always been evidence based in contrast to other systems of medicine which were not so evidence based. For a drug to be termed as effective a randomised control peer reviewed trial wouid have to be necessary Several cases are there in history of drugs being introduced and later withdrawn from the market either because of lack of effect or having serious side effects. In the case of Corona the speed at which the infections across the world left little time for mass studies A few multicentric studies highlighting use of hydroxychloroquine, Ivermectin, faviravir, dexamethasone were fast tracked and published in the highly respectable New England Journal of Medicine and The Lancet only to be withdrawn later perhaps being the only such papers to be withdrawn after publication. Others have tried using anti HIV drugs and plasma therapy for seriously ill patients. Some of these have been found to be successful. On the other side we have the Indian system of medicine that comes under AYUSH which stands for Ayurveda,Yoga, Unani, Siddha and Homeopathy. While technically Homepathy is not an Indian system of medicine having been propounded first by German Hahnemann it does gave a lot of practitioners in India. Once Corona cases started increasing there came report of a drug in homeopathy called Arsenic Album 18 which was supposed to cure Corona. I rang up one of my friends who is a homeopath to ask her about this drug. As luck would have it her husband had just recovered from Corona and she herself was not feeling too well. When I asked her about the medicine she said that her husband did have the medicine but the medicine was not a cure but just something to boost one's immunity much like the vitamins of modern medicine. Something similar was given in the Siddha system and distributed to everyone free of cost in Tamil Nadu.

In dengue for example a lot of people across the Indian subcontinent consume the extract of papaya or papaya juice In Indonesia I was told that it was guava juice. Again it is no sure but what it probably does is prevent the platelet count from dropping. In Ayurveda too, Yoga expert turned business man Baba Ramdev also tried to get approval from the health ministry for his Ayurveda medicine that was supposed to cure Corona but he got permission only to sell it as a immunostimulant. In neigbouring Sri Lanka also yet another indigenous practitioner Dhammika Bandara a carpenter by profession had thousands rushing to his house in Kegalle after he claimed that he had a syrup that could cure Corona He also offered the syrup to the Sri Lankan Health minister Pavithra Wanniarachi who took the syrup Subsequently the Ministry of health in Sri Lanka found that this syrup had no role in preventing the disease in treating it.

While modern medicine so far has no magic drug that will cure it and neither do the other systems of medicine it may be worthwhile taking a holistic view for treatment.

CHAPTER 20

How has India fared overall in the Corona epidemic.

India with a population of1380 million has presently about 10.2 million cases with about 1.47 lakh deaths.

In contrast USA with 330 million population has a total of about 18.8 million cases with about 3.3 lakh dead.

Brazil on the other hand with a population of 210 million has about 7.4 million cases with deaths amounting to 1.9 lakhs second only to USA It would appear that India has done fairly well in controlling the pandemic given its large population.

To recapitulate on the various salient features with some important questions which don't have ready answers.

1. How did the first person get the infection. Was it spread through bats or food from the sea food market?

2. Was it spread through other possible animals like snakes, pangolins, bats or pigs?

3. The mode of spread is droplet infection but the virus can also stay alive for varied time on surfaces like metals If that is the case will just social distancing and wearing masks alone help. Shouldn't then persons also wear gloves?

4. Thankfully children seem to be minimally affected and there is virtually no infant mortality due to Covid in hundreds of maybe thousand of cases one or other or both grandparents are affected and also parents but the child usually escapes even though sitting in the same house. Why?

The reason for this is not known while BCG vaccination given during infancy may give a protective effect with its efficacy This this has not been conclusively proven.

The comparison with Polio is interesting at this stage. Polio affects usually children and the route is feco oral route as a result of young children playing on the ground and then ingesting the polio virus. On the other hand children playing in exactly the same way do not get affected by the Corona virus. A rather interesting theory has come saying that the virus loses its intensity and becomes attenuated or less in intensity once it hits the ground.

4 Why hasn't it become a major health problem in the African continent which traditionally has been a hotbed for a number of diseases like Malaria HIV and relatively newer emerging diseases like Ebola West Nile fever etc. Obviously there may have had lesser air travel being largely poor countries and possibly fewer tests too. However no major lock-in was declared in most countries of Africa.

Could it be that Africans have some sort of immunity against Corona just like persons with Sickle cell trait in Africa have some immunity to malaria as is well documented?

Could there be something in the weather which may have reduced the virulence of the virus in some unknown way?

Another smaller example at home would be Bihar where one would have expected a number of cases the reality is that there are not many cases while Bihar did house to house survey early on in the program and also had plenty of awareness. It is still a mystery why the he numbers were so less It may be remembered that Bihar is one of India's most backward states and has traditionally been the home again of Malaria, Kalaazar, Polio. Not only just that they also become the first state to conduct a full fledged assembly election. As usual preceding the elections there were multiple rallies which did not adhere to covid protocol but nevertheless no major upsurge occurred in the number of cases.

So the question for the people of Bihar is the same as those for persons belonging to the African continent. Are the people of Bihar somewhat immune to Corona as compared to the rest of India.

Are they also somewhat immune to Corona by virtue of their being endemic for various other diseases.

5 How did the Southeast Asian countries do a much better job as compared to America and Europe. More specifically how did predominantly Buddhist countries like Cambodia, Vietnam, Laos and Myanmar do such a good job While definitely the experience of the SARS epidemic helped them, strict enforcing of social distancing rules and quarantine also helped. The Buddhist way of greeting Wai by rubbing the palms instead of a handshake also helped.

In many other South East Asian countries like Singapore countries it was already fairly common to see persons with masks much before corona.

6 Experts warn of a rise in winter in 2020 which may actually seem paradoxical because in winter generally the number of persons moving outdoors is much less. So does it mean that staying indoors can cause more infection?

7 Is use of airconditioners an increased risk for getting the Corona virus. Some articles published do not suggest so although conventional wisdom suggests that breathing in a closed space increases the risk a lot.

8 Do smog and stubble burning as practiced in many states particularly during winter increase the risk. Or would they actually drive out the virus.

India like the rest of the world also lost some celebrities due to Corona Among them was former President Pranab Mukherjee, popular playback singer SP Balasubramaniam who sang in several languages, Bengali veteran film actor Soumitra Chatterjee and highly respected Poetess Sugathakumari from Kerala.

CHAPTER 21

Where does one go from here. With cases going up particularly in Europe which expects a huge second wave in Winter it would be foolish to wait for herd immunity.

Obviously social distancing and wearing masks will have to be continued in 2021 also.

While schools will continue to remain shut for some more e time e learning will continue.

There will be restrictions on flights, Hotel bookings, gatherings including educational institutions and many other things for now.

While some countries like UK have started a second lockdown others like India don't seem to be in favour of it. In USA for example which went through a very hectic election campaign and more interesting no holds barred election hundreds of persons were seen in TV not wearing masks and not maintaining social distancing. Today USA again had a huge number of cases.

On the vaccine front news has been mixed. While some trials have had to be withdrawn citing adverse effects some have shown great promise In UAE for example vaccine had been introduced and the first person to take it was the ruler of UAE. In Russia also the vaccine has reportedly successful Chinese vaccine trials are indeed going in many countries. Yet another one done by Pfizer shows a lot of promise but it has a major technical problem in that it had to be stored at -70 degrees something which even highly advanced USA cannot have in most places.

As Dr Tedros of WHO mentioned it is better to have a universal Corona vaccine policy for all countries rather than having each country promote any one type of vaccine. However many countries are against this and they naturally want to be ahead in the race and roll out the vaccine faster and more effective. Obviously that is going to take time.

Regarding treatment there are so many regimens used by various states and countries most of which have not been per peer reviewed double blind Studies published in prestigious journals like The Lancet, New England Journal of Medicine have subsequently been forced to retract it The role of drugs like hydoxychloquuine ivermection, Dexamethasone, Faviparir etc at best remain debatable.

Coming to the vaccine while many vaccine companies are claiming success they have to be compared.

Vaccination had always been an intriguing story Right from the very first vaccination of Joseph Meissner by Louis Pasteur way back in 1885 technology developed so also newer vaccines. Take the case of the first vaccine against rabies first introduced by Louis Pasteur who used spinal tissue from rabid rabbits. He had earlier successfully tried it on rabid dogs. This nerve tissue vaccine though subsequently purified had severe neurological side effects and while it was used even till the eighties in India it was soon phased out Instead first a much costlier Human Diploid cell vaccine came followed by Chick and Duck embryo vaccine and Vero cell culture vaccines (cultured on monkey cells) that were free of side effects.

However even as vaccines are being developed for diseases like Corona there are some questions that are posed by the anti vaccine lobby that constitute a large number across the world. For example we have vaccines against a number of diseases but not one against malaria although the disease has been there for years. Yes vaccine trials are now on in 3 African countries but the question remains why is there not much excitement or hype for a vaccine that kills people each year.

Similarly the case of HIV vaccine While HIV was thought to be a killer disease in the eighties and nineties safe sex practices brought about a significant reduction in the number of cases and while work is going on for a vaccine against HIV it is no longer a priority.

And then there are are anti Vaxxers or the anti vaccine brigade a motley group that has over the years discredited vaccines all over the world.

One such myth that was propounded in India and elsewhere was regarding the oral polio vaccine or OPV that was supposed to make persons sterile. This took years to get rid of this wrong misconception. Once Wild polio virus 2 was eradicated in the world India started using Monovalent Oral polio vaccine for quite a while. Since it was found that majority of cases were due to type 1 wild polio virus over which the trivalent.

vaccine containing all 3 strains i.e Virus 1, 2 and 3 did not seem to have an effect monovalent OPV referred to as mOPV was introduced.

Ths led to another round of nonsense from the anti vaccine lobby saying the m referred to

Muslims and this was a special vaccine targeting the Muslims who seemed to have a high fertility rate Another issue that some raised was the presence of pork products in some of the vaccines This was never a concern much in India but it indeed was a concern in Muslim countries like Indonesia and Malaysia who wanted a Halal vaccine.

Perhaps the biggest misinformation regarding vaccination has been the role of MMR vaccination and its so called association with Autism. After initial publication in a few papers the iz was subsequently labeled as a fake association but by then the damage had been done.

Very recently the Brazilian president Bolsano has hit out against the Pfizer vaccinisne saying that the company takes no responsibility of side effects saying that women may grow a beard and voices could change after taking the vaccine a totally bizarre claim.

No vaccine can be termed hundred percent safe Many have small insignificant side effects like pain and swelling at the site of injection, induration or hardening of the area.

In more severe cases there is lymphodanopathy or swelling of the lymph glands. Most of these are known side effects and disappear very fast with treatment. What is more important is the possibility of any side effects that occur much later. It is of course very difficult to prove that a disease or syndrome was caused by administering a particular vaccine. A person for example could be diagnosed with say cancer or some other medical condition and if he has had a history of immunisation it would be wrong to impute his present condition to the vaccination. I n all such cases obviously the benefits exceed the risks. For example if 1lakh people take a vaccine and are protected against a disease but only 10 develop serious side effects it is definitely worth taking the risk.

The mRNA vaccine that has been developed by Pfizer seems the most promising and several countries havd rolled out their vaccines including USS, UK.

The m stands for messenger and RNAis an abbreviation of Ribonucleic acid. What exactly does this vaccine do Once injected into muscle it contains genetic instructions for making SARS Covv2 spike protein that is found on the surface of the virus causing Covid 19.This in turn triggers an antibody response that happens because the human cells do not recognize this.

Contrary to some myths mRNA vaccine dies not use a live virus.

Also it never enters DNA or Deoxyribonucleic acid which forms the basis of our genes Also the cells breaks down fast getting rid of mRNA.

There are also other questions like how many vaccines does an individual need.

How many doses of vaccine should India get assuming its just 2 dose per person.

Do we need to vaccinate the 1250 million population.

Ideally we should start with health workers and persons at risk.

If a vaccine plant has production of 1 million dose per month it will take more than 2 years to vaccinate everybody in India.

Also since the disease doesn't seem to affect children much. Can this wide group be dropped for the time being In that case the beneficiaries would be around 100 million?

And what about the cost. Assuming a cost of Rs 500 for the vaccine or about 8 dollars the total. Most for the vaccine alone would be 800 million dollars.

Most recently a participant in a trial claimed that he suffered severe neurological damage during the trial and has demanded compensation to the tune of Rs 5 crores from the vaccine manufacturers The vaccine manufactures on the other hand have slapped a case of defamation against the participant.

The health minister from the Haryana in India was given a shot in a double blind study by Bharat Biotechnology a company which is on the way to manufacturing one of the vaccines in production. However he developed Corona as per his own statement. This however led to the question as to whether he received the vaccine or a placebo meaning a similar sort of drug but which is harmless and has no protective use. But detractors point to the fact that media reports show him as getting the vaccine and not the placebo. This led to the company issuing a statement saying that the full effect is known only after getting a second dose and that after 45 days which theoretically meant that even after getting one shot or even two the protection may not be enough.

On the 8th of December 91 year old Margaret Keenan of UK became the first person in the world to get the approved vaccine This was produced by Pfizer and hundreds of persons have been vaccinated in the drive that began in UK.

Another patient who got the vaccine had an interesting name William Shakespeare. He too was a senior citizen.

The first shot of Corona vaccine in US was given on 14th December to health care workers from New York Sandra Lindsey who works as a registered nurse in Long Island Jewish Medical centre.

Subsequently FDA USA approved the use of Moderna vaccine giving Americans the choice of 2 vaccines Pfizer and Moderna. Later on President elect Joe Biden and Vicd president Elect Kamala Harris were also given the vaccine.

More recently England started vaccinating using the Oxford Asta Zeneca vaccine. India is also planning to do so shortly.

However there are ominous trends. A new variant of the Corona virus has been detected in UK which is far more contagious than the existing one. This has prompted UK to enforce a lockdown in almost half the country. Another such strain has been found in South Africa one of the worst hit African Nations with a tally of over 8 lakh cases. As a result of the panic button pressed by UK many countries across the world have stopped their flights to and from UK temporarily.

It is hoped that these new strains which may be more contagious would however not be more lethal. The mutant strain has already reached several countries including Singapore, Italy, and India.

One hopes that 2021 will see the whole world vaccinated and effectively kill this pandemic.

www.ingramcontent.com/pod-product-compliance
Lightning Source LLC
Chambersburg PA
CBHW051259250726
48656CB00004B/1369